Wounded, But Not Broken

The Life of a Therapeutic Foster Child

ANGEL BARTLETT

ILLUSTRATED BY: TONI THORNE

authorHOUSE

AuthorHouse™
1663 Liberty Drive
Bloomington, IN 47403
www.authorhouse.com
Phone: 1-800-839-8640

© 2010 Angel Bartlett. All rights reserved.

No part of this book may be reproduced, stored in a retrieval system, or transmitted by any means without the written permission of the author.

First published by AuthorHouse 08/12/2010

ISBN: 978-1-4520-5406-3 (e)
ISBN: 978-1-4520-5405-6 (sc)
ISBN: 978-1-4520-5404-9 (hc)

Library of Congress Control Number: 2010910459

Printed in the United States of America

This book is printed on acid-free paper.

I dedicate this book to the thousands of abused and abandoned children in foster care who will never have a place to call home. I am your voice, and I know your pain. But if you continue to pursue your dreams and aspirations, you will accomplish the great goal that God has set forth for you, because he knows your beginning and end. To the kids in detention, group homes, and even those who are homeless, I have not forgotten about you. You must channel your anger and your depression to help you push forward to something that is much greater than your current situation. Always remember, what does not kill you will only make you stronger! At times you may feel weak, but God will never put more on you than you can bear! I am not telling you what I think; I am speaking to what I know! Do not give up on yourself. Your past does not determine your future! They once called me "a menace to society" they told me "I would never make it" they counted me out. The same people that judged me and labeled me are now my colleagues. We may not always understand the valleys and we may surely not like them, but trust the process! God has never failed. ***"Before I formed you in the wound I knew you, before you were born I set you apart; I appointed you as a prophet to the nations"! (Jeremiah 1:5)***

Angel Bartlett Wins Spirit of Youth Award
VJJA Assists with Scholarship

Angel Bartlett, 26, of Hampton, was presented with the Virginia Advisory Committee on Juvenile Justice's 2008 Virginia Spirit of Youth Award. The award was presented in conjunction with the 2008 *Making a Difference in Juvenile Justice* Conference in June. In addition to the award, Angel was also presented with an educational scholarship. The Virginia Juvenile Justice Association (VJJA) was among the donors.

Modeled after the National Coalition on Juvenile Justice's Spirit of Youth Award, the Virginia Spirit of Youth Award recognizes and celebrates a young adult, under the age of 28, who has made great strides following involvement with the juvenile justice system; has overcome personal obstacles; and is making significant contributions to society. The award is it its third year in Virginia. Previous Virginia winners have included Forrest Perry of Rocky Mount and Marvin Gumba of Norfolk. (Read about Forrest in our archives at: www.vjja.org/eAdvocate/Summer2007).

Angel was nominated for the award by VJJA President Beth Stinnett, Hampton Juvenile & Domestic Relations Court Judge Jay Dugger and Deputy Director of Hampton Human Services Wanda Rogers. A former foster care child, probationer, and resident of Bon Air Juvenile Correctional Center, Angel is now a college graduate, a full-time government employee, a full-time graduate student, a homeowner, a biological parent and a foster care parent.

Through her work as a Family Crisis Stabilization Worker at the Hampton Department of Human Services, Angel has become a dedicated and vocal advocate for children in both the dependency and delinquency systems. She and her colleagues work closely with the staff at the Hampton Court Service Unit to ensure that children from families in crisis do not enter secure detention by default when detention would not have been indicated by the seriousness of the charge. Instead workers respond on-site and children and families are offered intensive services and respite. Angel is proud to be employed in a position in which she can have a direct impact on children and families and prevent children with circumstances similar to her own from being removed from their families and penetrating deeper into the delinquency system.

In her letter supporting Angel's nomination, Deputy Director Rogers said, "I first met Angel at a Juvenile Justice Conference where she served on a youth panel. I remember Angel talking about being in foster care and how the separation from her family made her feel. She also talked about her involvement in the juvenile justice system. She reflected on her anger and turmoil as she tried to navigate the foster care system and the juvenile justice system. It was very difficult and at times she felt very lonely. I am especially proud that Angel did not give up. Approximately two years ago I was again face-to-face with Angel. This time I was welcoming her as a newly selected social worker at the Hampton Department of Human Services. Despite the obstacles Angel has faced she is an amazing example of the potential that lies within so many of the youth we serve. As I listen to her talk I can hear the determination that she has to help anyone who crosses her path. She has chosen not to be bitter about her circumstances but rather to use them to help others".

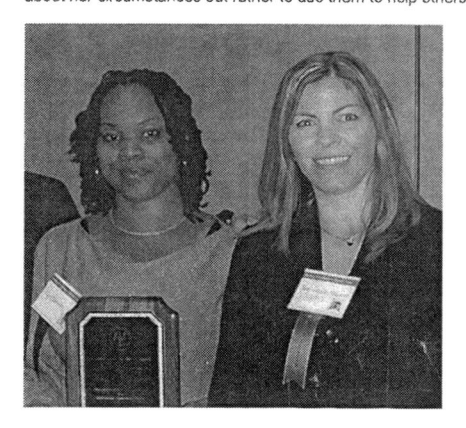

As I sit alone thinking of the right words to say, I think, *Where do I begin?* I wonder how I can put my chaotic life on paper. It is my belief that my life is a living testimony and that I was created to break the yoke and devour strongholds. I question how do I begin to express who I am, and why I am passionate about families, foster parents, and more important, the thousands of children who are displaced every day because of parental incarceration, substance abuse, physical abuse, neglect, sexual exploitation and thousands of other reasons. I think about my life and how I never had the opportunity to be a child that experienced the love of family. I think about the moments that were stolen from an innocent girl, and my heart begins to beat faster and faster, and the tears begin to formulate in my eyes. I have been writing this book about my life for several years, but each time I have attempted to write it, I get writer's block, or is it the pain of putting it on paper? Is it the fear of people judging me? Or is it yet another trick of the enemy to keep me from my destiny? Or is it just the indolent and depressing spirit that still lives in me?

So, I will first start with acknowledging the devil, you have lost again and as I write and push through the tears I am secretly laughing at you because you can't do anything to God's chosen vessel. So my recommendation is to get your hands off me! I am the "SERVANT

JOB" in the new millennium! Take everything that I have, but you cannot stop DESTINY! "HAHAHAHA" ***"For he wounds, but he also binds up; he injures, but his hands also heal". (Job 5:18)***

To all the influential people who have made such a great impact on my life, be it positive or negative. I want to thank my biological mother and father for bringing me into this world. There was one time in my life when I hated you both and would not have dared uttered a word even to mention that you exist. But, through God, I have truly learned how to forgive; but I will never forget! Even though life was hell, I can say that my life lessons have only made me stronger, and I vow every day to give my daughter so much more than what was given to me!

I have had more than a dozen placements in the course of my lifetime: foster-care placements, detention homes, group homes, extended family members. I never had a place to call home, but through it all, I have survived and I am still standing! *Wounded, but not broken.*

I thank all the people who have supported me when I did not believe in myself. To my mom (RIP) Gwendolyn Tose Rigell, even though I did not share your blood, you were by far the best thing that ever happened to me. I will always carry you in my heart and soul and continue to reach a level of success that you always told me that I was capable of obtaining! There will never be enough words to describe how much I miss you and desire for you to be here in my life! "Momma, "I am still struggling to find my way, I am still learning how to love and how to be loved. I am still struggling with pain and the search for my true identity and I need you to help guide me and keep me sane." She would say, "I am always here," but it's just not the same and it never will be. Thank you for loving me when I did not know how to love myself! I dedicate this book to you!

To Pastor Eddie (RIP), thank you for laying my foundation and teaching me that without God there is no such thing as true peace! You always told me that the devil wanted to keep me bound so that I would not be able to be a part of change, but I am no longer in bondage, and I thank you for the seeds that you have planted in me. You have left me "well able and well equipped." You will always be missed, and I thank you for loving me!

To Mom Pettaway, thank you for being tough, sometimes too tough, but it's a cold world, and we all need a little tough love! Thank you for seeing me through and always having my back. I love you dearly. You are the craziest white woman ever; the Most High blessed me with you and dad!

To my daughter, Malana Jules LaVille, you are the air that I breathe. I never knew love until I knew you. I strive so hard to be the perfect mother, but I know I have my faults. When you read this book, I want you to know your mother struggles, but despite what life placed upon me, I am a survivor and so are you, my dear child. Momma loves you, but remember God loves you more. I pray that I will always be an example before you and that you will grow up in the fear and ammunition of the Most High.

To all the foster parents who I have given hell, and all the foster parents currently going through hell while trying to parent children who are broken, I say thank you. To the judges, guardian-Ad-litem, counselors, teachers, social workers, and probation officers, I say thank you.

To all the people who said that I would never make it, abused and misused me, **read the book**, I am still here and stronger than ever! Oh, and this is only the beginning, because I am going to take the world by storm for I am more than a conqueror.

The Angel's in my life
An Angel is defined as "a messenger of God a person regarded as beautiful, good, and innocent". God placed specific Angel's in my life to help me find my way and to pray for me when I did not know how to pray…. I will never forget my Angel's and I am forever grateful.

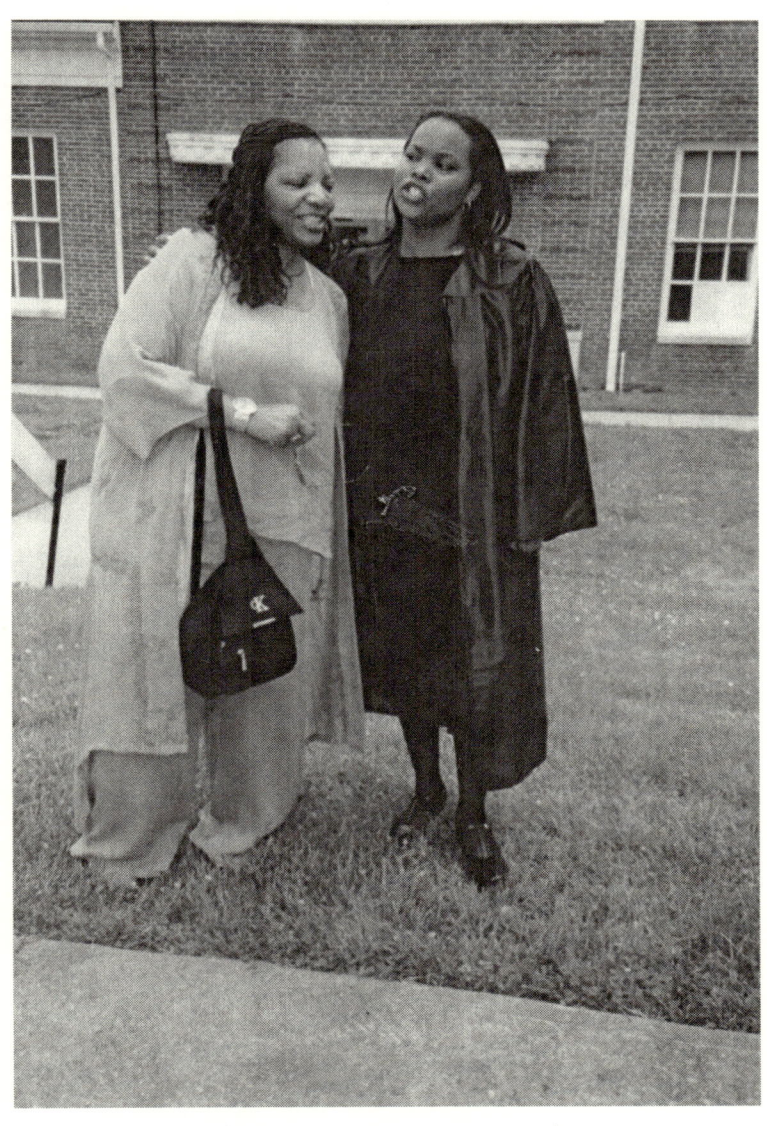

*Me and Mom Gwen at my 2003 graduation.
Too know her was to love her.*

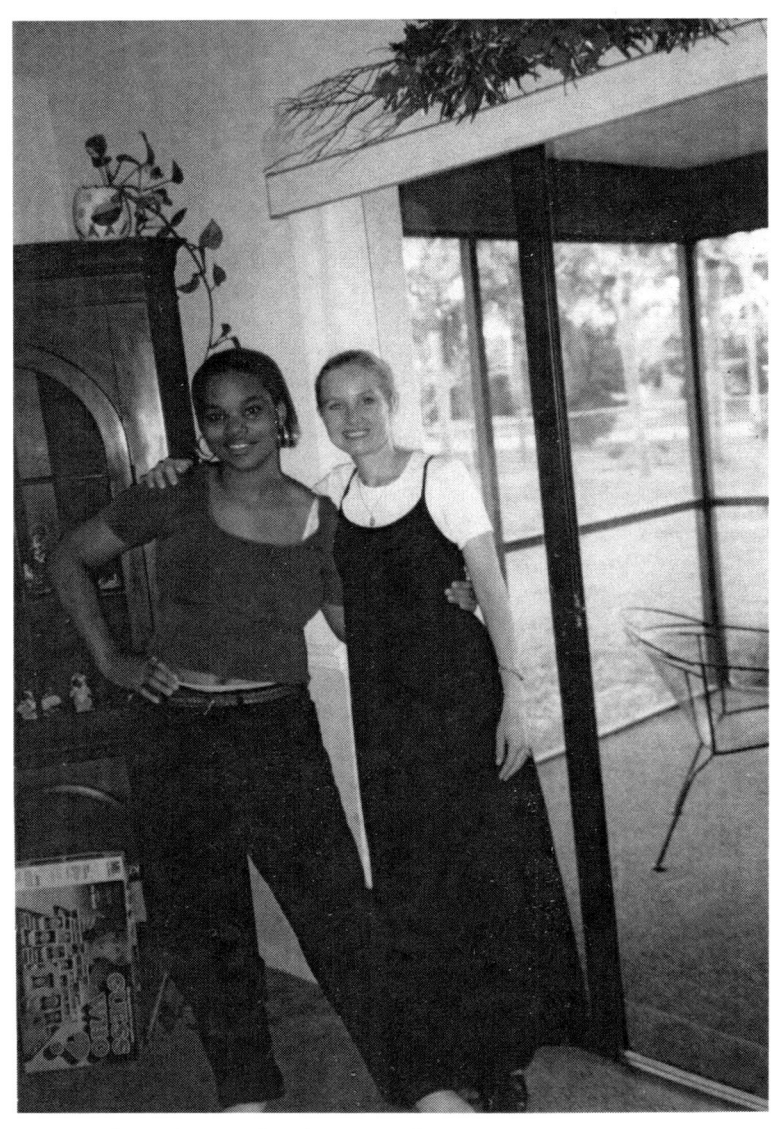

My Social Worker in Florida. Ms.Kellie Menke she inspired me greatly.

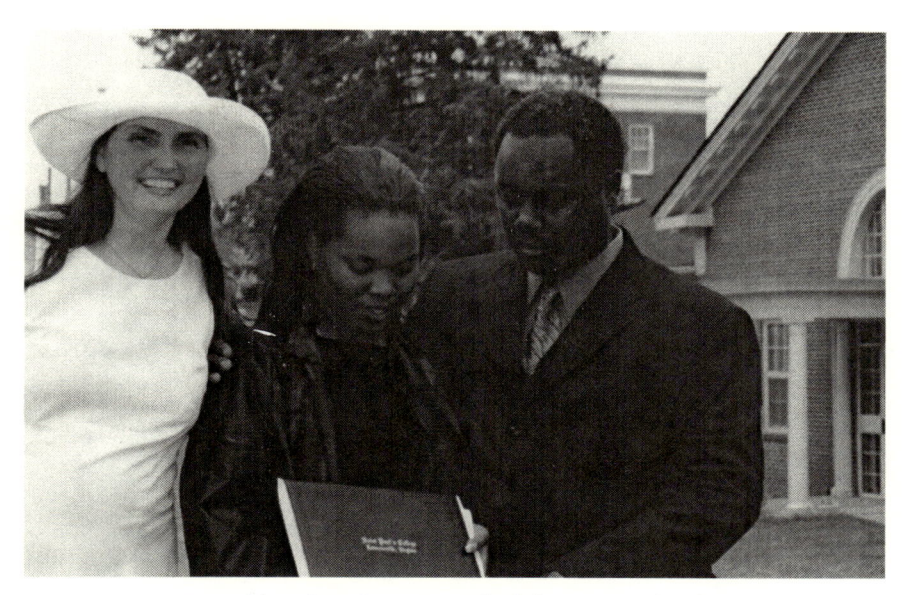

*I was blessed with two wonderful moms and a dad.
What the devil meant for me not to have God doubled it and gave me two!*

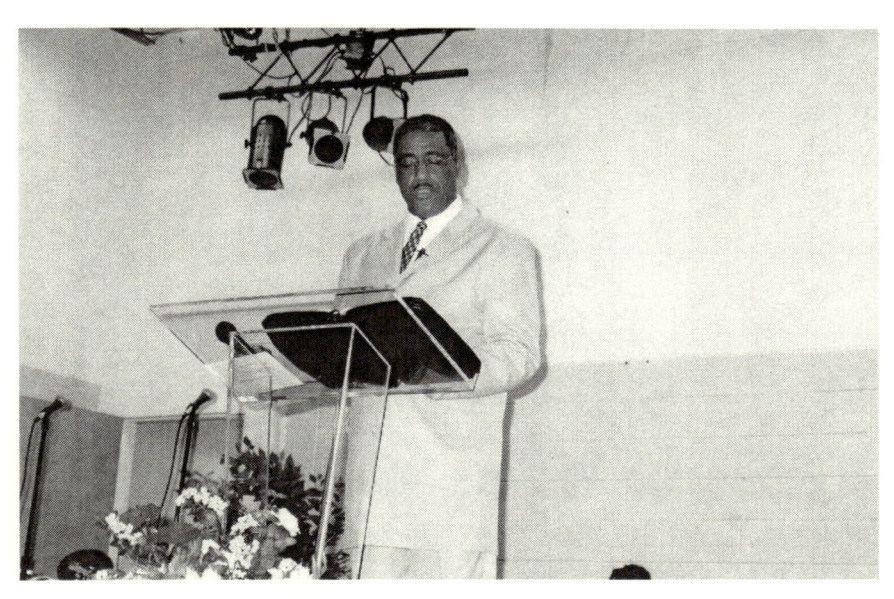

*The late great Pastor Eddie Clemons and founder of Resurrection House. The
seed was already planted, but I thank you for everything that you birthed in me!
I am finally out of the box!*

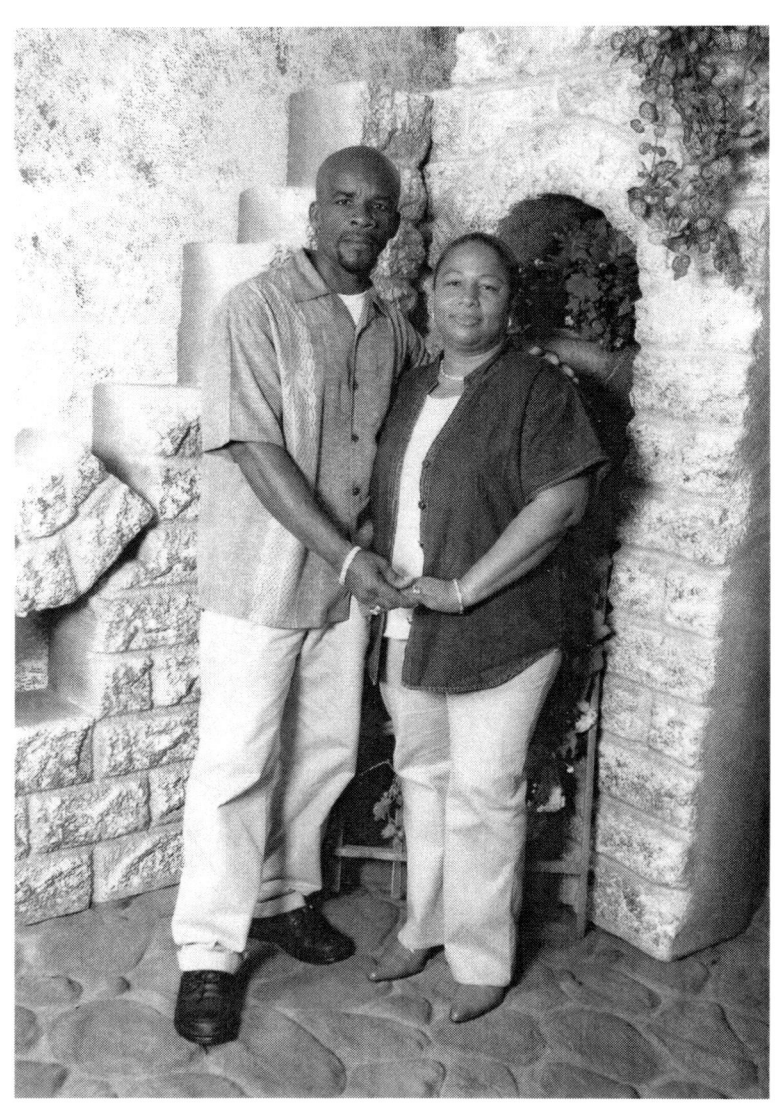

My daughter's paternal grandparents. Malana is blessed to have what I never had and her grandparent's help create a big part of the story! I love them for loving my daughter and being the best grandparents anyone could ever ask for.

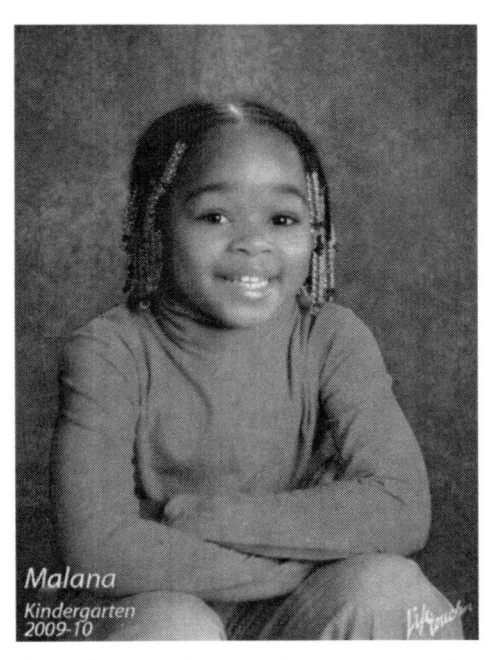

The best thing that ever happened to me, next to being saved!

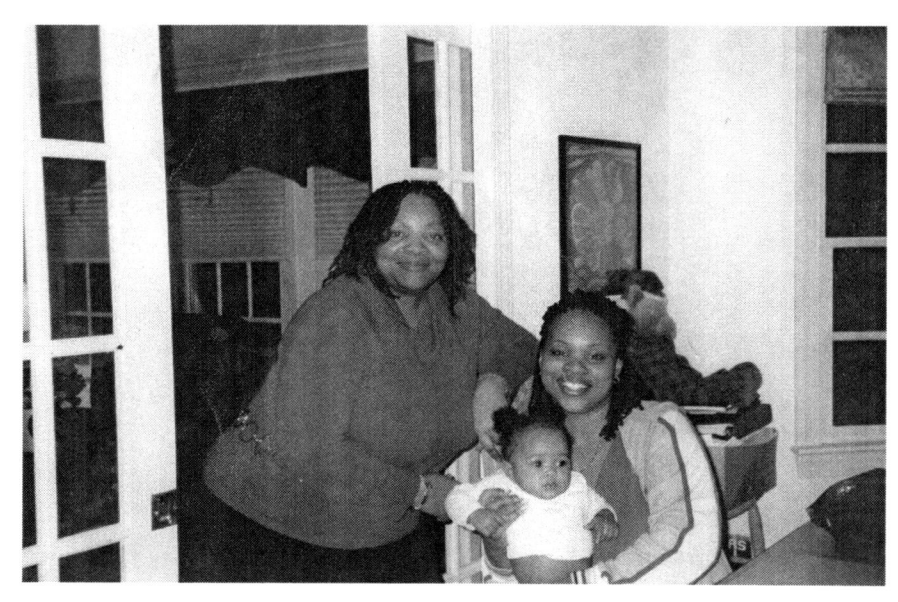

Mom Gwen, me and Malana

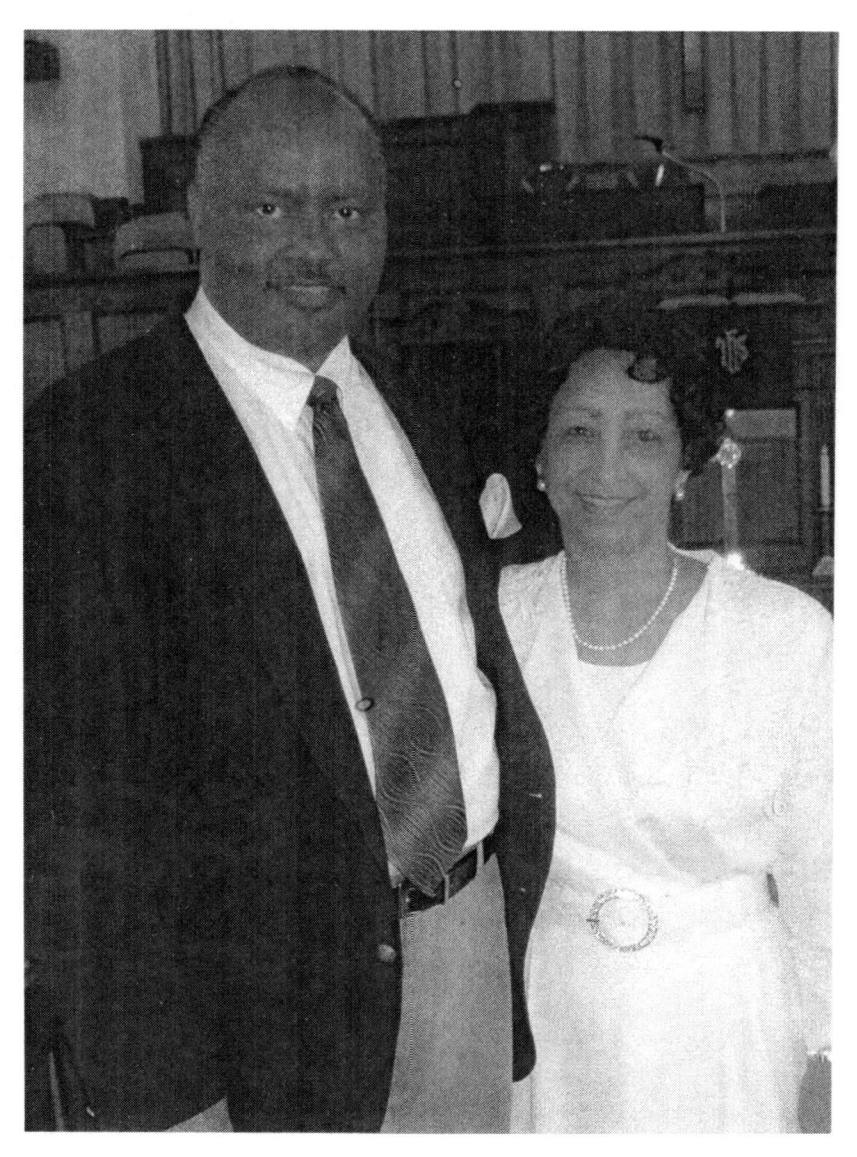

Always made me feel right at home and has always been in my corner.

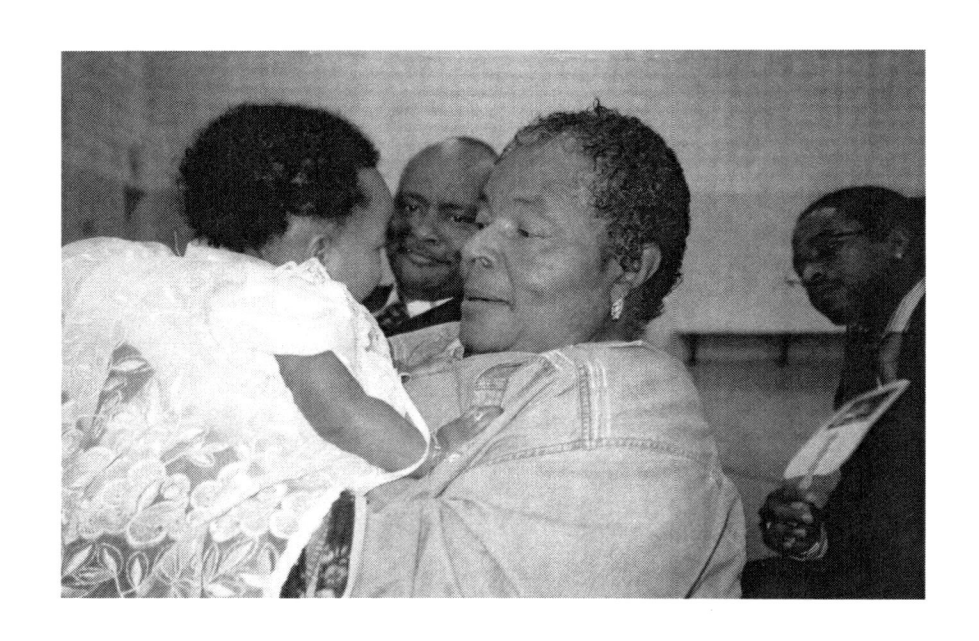

Daisy
Thank you for raising five great children and accepting me as your crazy granddaughter.

Still Standing

I was born in 1981 in Newport News Hospital. I imagine when I was born I was a happy baby. My dad named me Angel, because he said that I was his little angel. I had an older sister, who was two years older than I. I don't remember much about our childhood, so I will start where I can remember the most.

I never knew the reason that my sister and I began living with our paternal grandparents. I don't recall ever being with my mother when I was a baby. I do remember her coming to visit us and bringing nice things: clothes, shoes, and candy. Every time she left, I would run down the driveway, tears streaming down my eyes, saying, "Mommy, please don't go. Come back, I want to go with you!" Whenever I had a visit with my mom, my whole attitude would change. I would be very mean to my grandparents, because I thought they were the ones who were keeping us from living with our mother. I would see the hurt on my grandparents' faces, but they would always console me. It was though my grandmother wanted to tell me the entire story, but she could not bring herself to hurt my heart. So she would just allow me to sob and comfort me when she could. I never understood why months would go by without seeing my mom, but no matter how long the day or the hour,

I longed to have her in my life. It's funny, because I still have that same feeling this day. It's called a child's love for her mother.

I remember my sister would always say, "Stop crying, girl. She doesn't want us, and we have a good home." Even though my sister and I had different emotions as it related to our mother, she would always make me feel better. But she did not like me disrespecting our grandparents, and she made that well known to me. On the weekends, we would always go and see Dad. At the time, I did not know that dad was in the penitentiary, serving a six-year bid for strong-armed robbery. Kids can believe the dumbest things. I always thought Dad was at this fun camp, and I cried and held onto the fences every time we left. I remember going through the gates and being checked by security and wondering why they always took the good food that we brought for Dad. "Mean guards": I thought they just want to eat it themselves!

We had so much fun on each visit, playing hopscotch, double Dutch, pin the tale on the donkey! I hated leaving my dad behind those wires, and I only wanted him to come home. I had no idea he was locked up; I always thought that he stayed because he wanted to. I looked forward to seeing my father every weekend.

One day, I held onto the fence and cried my eyes out. "Daddy, please come home, please don't stay here!" My grandfather was pulling me, and my grandmother said if I did not stop, I could not come and visit again. I cried the entire way home, and again, big sister was always there to console me. I never understood why everyone else had a mom and dad, and we only had Grandma and Grandpa. I mean, they were great and took excellent care of us, but I wanted a momma and daddy. My dad would always tell me that he was coming soon and that we would be a family again. The sad part was that I never remembered us being a family. I always knew us to live with our grandparents. I always anticipated the day that Dad would come home. I dreamed of us packing our bags and me, my sister, and my mom being this big, happy family. That was my daily prayer.

The visits with my mom continued, and even though they were sporadic, I looked forward to each and every visit. I don't remember the day Dad came home, and I don't remember how old I was, but it was the happiest day of my life, I think. I don't recall Dad always staying with us at Grandma and Granddad's. But I remember he often took us out to the movies. He called my sister Bonehead #1, and I was Bonehead #2. Daddy was always doing fun things with us. He adored his girls. Sometimes he would come to the house, and he would smell funny and be acting real silly. At the time, I did not know that Daddy was drunk as hell. I would often hear Grandpa and Grandma telling him that he was not going to keep coming around with that foolishness and confusing us girls. I can remember running into the kitchen and saying, "Please don't make Daddy go away." Daddy said something really stupid, and I was told to go upstairs. I went upstairs weeping, and I heard my granddaddy smack the snot out of my dad! From there, I don't know what happened, because I closed my door and wept in my bed. We never got to spend time with Mom and Dad together, and Dad always avoided the question. Whenever I asked my mom, she would say that things did not work out with them, because they were from two different worlds and my dad was an alcoholic. She told me that I was too young to understand. The visits with my mom and dad went on for several years. As we got older, my grandmother would make us spend more time at our aunt's house, and I hated going there, because my uncle was very mean to us and treated us differently than he treated his own kids. I remember sitting at his kitchen table one day, and he had fixed me a sandwich and put mayonnaise on it. He knew that I did not like mayonnaise, but he told me that I was not going to eat a dry sandwich in his house. I told him the sandwich was not dry to me, but he said, "Don't you talk back to me," and smacked me in my face and told me that I was going to sit there until I ate the sandwich. I cried profusely and then he came and began to smash the sandwich in my mouth and tell me how I was not his responsibility, and I needed to be with my momma, instead of giving them a headache and running up their bills. I sat at the table for hours before he finally let me get up before my aunt came home. He told me to go and clean up and that I better not ask for anything to eat and not to say anything to my aunt. I always wondered how my aunt, being so sweet, could be with such a mean man. I don't think she had a clue as to how he treated me and my sister, but I dared not say one word! I was tired of staying with them and wanted to go back with my grandparents. One day, I called my grandma and begged to come home, and that is when the talk came.

It was after church one Sunday, and my grandma and granddad called us in the living room and sat us down. They said that Grandma had been sick and that they were going to allow us to start spending some weekends, and maybe Christmas, with our mom. I told my grandma that I no longer wanted to stay with my aunt and uncle, but they said that we had no choice, because our dad was not able to take care of us, and they needed help in raising us. So I asked why could we not go and stay with our mom permanently. My grandfather responded by saying, "Angel, be careful what you ask for." My grandfather told me to be thankful that we would be allowed to spend weekends and holidays, but I just did not understand. So I decided to just take advantage of the time that we would begin to have with my mom. I wanted to know how soon we would be able to begin our visits. My grandma forced a smile and said next weekend. This was very exciting for me. My grandma told us that if anyone ever tried to hurt us to make sure that we told them immediately. I wondered why Grandma said this. I never knew the whole story as to what led us to live with our grandparents, but I guess it was not good. My mom always told us that when my dad went to jail she was not financially able to take care of us.

When the visits begin to take place, everything was going really good. My sister never showed any emotions when it came to Mom or Dad. Dad was always in and out of our life, but I knew he did not like us having the visits with Mom. Mom had a boyfriend and a son by this man, but from what I could tell, everything was fine. Dad was always telling us that he was working, trying to get his own place, so he could give us a home, but he was always doing disappearing acts. When it was time to return from our weekend visits, I would cry and beg Momma not to take us back, but she would always tell me one day soon we would all be together.

It's amazing how a person can be on drugs, but you never notice anything about their behavior. Because you love them so much, you look past all their imperfections, and you only want to be loved and accepted by them ... **The strength of a mother's love and the daughters who longed to be loved by their mothers.**

I Finally Got My Wish

One Sunday, we came home from a visit with our mom, and again, I cried and chased the car down the drive way because I did not want her to leave. When I finally got done crying my eyes out and lying out in the driveway, I made my way to the house. My grandparents were sitting in the living room with my sister, and my grandmother had a look of worry on her face. My grandfather told me to take a seat, and so I did. This conversation changed my life forever. My grandfather started by saying that my grandmother has been really sick and had several strokes. My sister was crying, and I was just looking puzzled. My grandmother began saying how she loved us dearly but that she understood that we wanted to be with our mother. She said, "I don't want you all to go, but maybe it will be best, because my health is declining." My grandfather said that they would always be there, but at the end of the school year, we would be going to live with our mother in King and Queen. I was sad that my grandmother was not feeling well but elated that I was finally going to get to live with my mother. After all, my dad's visits were getting fewer by the weeks.

My sister continued to weep, and as we went to our room upstairs, I said, "Peaches, why are you crying? We get to go and live with Momma."

She just looked at me and said, "Girl, Momma doesn't want us for real!" I immediately got angry and said, "Yes she does. You'll see!" The next visit with Momma I was so happy. She smiled and said, "I told you I would bring my girls home!" I asked her if we would still see our dad, and she said yes, we would be allowed to see him whenever we wanted. While living with my grandparents, we lived in a big house, but my mom lived in a little three-bedroom trailer, but it did not matter to me. It was a major change, but I thought as long as I was with Momma, nothing else mattered. The visits with Momma became much easier, because I knew that time was winding down before we would be with her permanently. When she dropped us off, I would be on my best behavior and never cried. Our dad made it known that he was not happy about the decision for us to go and live with our mom. He asked why we did not want to live with our aunt and uncle, and I quickly told him that Uncle Pick was evil, and I told him what he did that day with the sandwich. My dad had tears in his eyes and asked me why I never told. I told him that I was afraid and thought no one would believe me. I also told him about the smack. My dad was furious, but I told him if we could not live with him, I only wanted to go home to Momma. I talked with him about my feelings and how I felt when I saw other kids with their moms and dads. He told me that he understood and apologized for not being a better dad. I told him it was okay and that in my eyes he was the best! My dad tried to talk to my sister about her feelings, but she never shared much; she only told my dad that she did not care where we lived.

Be Careful What You Wish For!

Well, I don't remember exactly the date or the time of the transition, but it appeared to happen fast, immediately after we got out of school. Saying good-bye to my grandparents was hard, and saying good-bye to my cousins was even harder, but I was so happy to finally be with my mom. I remember the first night we got to the trailer, something felt strange. I guess it was the idea of knowing that I was not going back to my grandparents. We went from a big two-story house to a small three-bedroom trailer. It wasn't long before I began noticing things about my mom.

The first thing I noticed was her irritability. Those weekend visits always were pleasant, but when she had to deal with us on a full-time basis, she didn't have much patience! She worked us like slaves, and while we were use to chores, we were not use to having to be responsible for doing so much and taking care of our little brother. She was always arguing with my brother's father, and it was often about us; we would listen to them at night. My sister and I were not familiar with domestic violence, but we quickly learned. It amazed me how things took a turn for the worst so quickly, and as things took a turn, so did my feelings. I was not use to aggressive behavior and definitely did not know how to respond to it. But this was frequent in our new placement with our mom. I had heard her curse on a few occasions and she would always apologize, but as time progressed the curse words became more frequent and were eventually directed towards us. It seemed as though she was angry with us because we came to live with her. She began to leave us by ourselves at night for long periods of time. We were not use to this, and I often found myself crying on my sister's shoulder. I tried so hard to please my mom and to make things the way they use to be, but no matter how hard I tried, things continued to get worse. We had no structure. Our brother would be with his dad, and his dad would bring him to the house when he needed a babysitter. We often went without food, and we had no real idea of how to cook because at Grandma's, the meals were always prepared.

I remember my sister would look at me, roll her eyes, and say, "I told you she did not want us." I use to weep in the bed for hours, wondering what was happening to our life. My mom's boyfriend was nice, but only when he needed a favor for his son! His son was always well taken care of. I felt as though I was living in a different country. I longed to go back home to my grandparents. When it was time to start school, my brother had gone school shopping and received several new outfits. When I asked my mom about our clothes, she would talk about my dad being a deadbeat and how she could not afford to buy us clothes. She would say very evil things about our grandparents and how we were little spoiled brats! I would look at my mom and have total disbelief in my eyes. I can actually remember having a pain in my heart, because this was not what a mother was supposed to be. My grandparents never treated us this way. I will never forget the first time I saw my mom get hit by my brother's father. I was terrified; they fought as though they were two men in the streets. We would often hear them fight, but witnessing it was a different type of trauma. When it was all over, we were made to clean up the mess and told that it best be clean when she got home. She had no concern for our feelings or how terrified we were after seeing this. He left with his son, and she left right behind him. It did not take long before we realized that the two of them fighting was normal. I never got use to it, and I cried every time. Eventually, the beatings and the name-calling would begin with us. It was nothing for her to say, "Come here, you little bitch." She spoke to us as though we were not her daughters. It seemed as though the very sight of us made her sick. She would come home late at night and always wake me up to scratch her back, rub her feet or fix her something to drink. It never mattered if I had school the next morning. She picked on me far more than my sister, and I took this to be because I was the weak one who was always crying. My sister, on the other hand, never said much, and it took a lot to make her cry. However, I cried enough tears for the both of us. Life was beginning to feel like hell. This woman, who I thought that I had loved so much and who loved me, had turned into a total stranger. But she never spoke to our brother the way that she talked to us. I think I cried myself to sleep every night.

As time progressed, I learned that everyone in this family was dysfunctional. I began to spend more time with some of my aunts and my maternal grandmother. My grandmother was very strange and very evil. If I had to diagnose her, it would be with bi-polar. She could be very humble and sweet and then do a complete 360 on you minutes later and call you every name but a child of God! She and my mother did not get along and often had arguments. She would always tell us that we should have stayed with our grandparents, because our mom was no good and was a crackhead! We never knew what a crackhead was, but we began to hear it quite frequently. And though I did not know what a crackhead was, my mom showed all the characteristics of someone that had some significant problems. So naturally, with time I came to understand that my mom was a crackhead, and that our family was greatly impacted by this drug. This made me observe her behavior even closer, because my grandma and other aunts were always talking about her. I thought, *I am living in hell*. I had crazy cousins, and people in the community were always making fun of me, because I was living in poverty and dressed like I was living in poverty. There was no hiding it. The kids at school were always making fun of me and my sister because my mom was always at the corner store begging for coins. I also later found out that she was a well known prostitute and often would trick to receive drugs. I hated having to go to Grandma's because she was also crazy and enjoyed beating me with an extension cord, but at Grandma's I always knew that I would never be hungry.

I hated living in King and Queen everyone knew that my mom was a crackhead and the kids were so mean to me. I remember the feeling of fear that would develop when I would see my mom, but also anger. I had been with my mom for several months, but I still was not use to this lifestyle, and I really felt with all my heart that no child should have to live a life full of hunger, beatings and abuse. The weekends that I remember having with my mother and the dreams of being a family where totally diminished! There were no fun times and I felt no love, just lots of anger and abuse that I had to endure. My dad was in and out of jail, and we never heard from our paternal grandparents or any of our paternal side of the family. It was as if we had become total strangers and we no longer existed.

I began to engage more with the community and often got into a little trouble in school. If I was with my grandmother and got suspended from school, I would surely get an extension cord on my ass. Grandma was serious about education, because she only went to the third grade and could not read. None of her children graduated from high school, and she was so disappointed with all of them. So when it came down to me, she didn't play when it came to school and I always had to read. If I struggled with a word she would beat me and tell me to study harder. But if it was up to my mom to discipline me when it came to my school work it would never happen, because she was never home or too high to do anything except sleep or look for her next fix. She would always tell me that I wasn't going to be anything in life so stop pretending. Even though I was now making poor choices and being severely abused and neglected, I always paid close attention to what my grandma said about babies and reading. So I knew I was not going to be another victim and have a baby, because I was afraid of sex my grandmother told me horror stories about how the dick can get stuck in your pussy and paralyze you.

She also told me that if my cherry was busted that I may never walk again. At the time I did not know any better so I believed her and was horrified to even look at a boy. I always read, because I was afraid of being a dummy and having to always live in poverty. So no matter what we were going through, I always made sure that I was reading and keeping my legs closed so that I would not get pregnant. Reading became my way to escape even though it was only for a little while.

Living in King and Queen, life was beginning to happen and my sister and I had to catch on fast. There were so many times that I can actually say that I wanted to commit suicide because life was just that bad. That was a very strong emotion to feel at such a young age, but so were hate and the feeling of being unloved. This was a culture shock for me. It speaks to the saying, "Every person, every season has its honeymoon stage." I had thought my mom was the greatest and was going to take excellent care of us, and I thought living in a trailer was going to be fine; but life was not fine. I was being introduced to life quickly. I went from being sheltered, having structure and being in church all the time to never attending church and never being supervised. From being taught to pray and read the Bible to how to steal and survive. We seldom saw our mom, and when we did, it was always a demand that we needed to do immediately or something we had to do for our brother. We never laughed or spent time together. She was always bringing men around us, and they would look at me like they really wanted to fuck me, my grandma had taught me about those looks. They were always old as hell, and the thought of their eyes on me made me sick! She seldom looked me in my eyes, and I believe it was because she was ashamed of herself. I had grown a hatred for my mother, and the very sight of her made me sick. A person should never feel that type of hatred, especially a child toward its mother.

I can remember as though it were yesterday, Mom telling me to get her some soda. I calculated my steps very closely. The first thought that came to mind was spitting in her can and then I thought, *Well, I can put a little bleach in it, and maybe she will die!* I was afraid that she was going to smell the bleach, but I did not care. I had to see if this would kill her. I knew that if she smelled it, she would beat the living shit out of me. An as I brought the drink to her, she looked at me and asked, "You wouldn't try to kill me, would you?" I was so shocked that she knew I hated her that much. I told her no, and she told me to drink out of the soda first. I hesitated, but only for one moment. If a sip did kill me, at least I would not have to deal with her anymore, and anything was better than living in this home. I took a sip and then gave it to her; she only drank a little. She had been gone for several days and just wanted sleep. I spent that whole evening waiting for her to die, but she never did. When we got up, she was gone. I told my sister what I did, and she just said, "Girl, you are lucky that she did not smell it." My own sister did not care if we killed our mom. I felt bad, because my sister had always warned me, and I was a little mad with her, because she always saw something about mom but never said what it was. But she had turned our lives upside down, and we only had each other. We had two pair of decent jeans, and our shoes were never the best. We had to hand wash our socks and panties each night and place them on the vents to dry so that we may have clean panties and socks for each day.

As time progressed, we got a little older and a lot wiser. We began to develop into young ladies, and this brought even more problems our way. I depended on my sister for everything. She was my protection, and even though we did not get along that well, she would fight a battle for me at the drop of a dime! My sister and I were always missing school. It was generally for lack of motivation, no clean clothes, or the trailer was so cold we could not move. We never knew when our mom would be at home, so there was no one to hold us accountable other than Grandma, and we tried to stay away from her because she was crazy.

One day we went to school and were called to the office. The school administrator told us that there was someone from social services who wanted to talk with us. This was my very first encounter with a social worker, but certainly not my last. She asked us several questions, and I told her everything she wanted to know with some additional information. I wanted to be rescued. Well, I guessed she finally caught up with my mom, and when she did, we were punished severely. I will never forget the look in my mom's face before she beat the living hell out of me and my sister. She said that we better tell that white bitch that everything we told her was a lie. I was so angry, and I felt betrayed. How could she tell my mom everything that I had disclosed? Didn't she know that she would beat us? She was suppose to rescue us, but instead she caused us more pain. She came back to school again, and I was rude as hell. I told her everything was a lie, and I was only seeking attention. I told her that our mom would not beat us and she was a good mom.

The abuse continued, and as my mom's drug habit grew hungrier, things got increasingly worse. I remember this man telling my mom that he wanted to dance with me, and in order for her to get a hit, I had to dance. At this point in my life, I was use to the unexpected. I had developed an attitude of what's next in life? As each day passed I was always introduced to something new I felt as though things could not get any worse so why not just go with the flow. I hated to dance with this man, but at this point, it was dance or fight. My mom enjoyed using me as her punching bag, and if I ever made her lose out on getting a fix, I was guaranteed to suffer from a few of her beatings. She told me to dance with him, because he was going to take us into to town later and buy us some stuff that we wanted to eat from the grocery store. I knew what that meant. That meant we would go to the grocery store and whatever steak was brought, she would cook it for my brother and his father, but me and my sister would eat whatever was left over if anything at all. But, as usual, I went along with the plan. I allowed this man to hold me close to his body as he caressed my back and whispered sweet nothings in my ear. My mom sat at the kitchen table and watched after she came out of the room from getting high. When the dance was over, I guess she got pissed because of how he was still looking at me. I had a fake ponytail piece in my hair, and she told me to take it out. I said that I would not, and as I began to walk away, rolling my eyes she punched me in my back so hard that I fell to the floor. She yanked the hair out of my hair and said, "Bitch, don't you ever walk away from me." The entire time, she pinched my cheeks as tight as she could, and tears were streaming down my eyes. I mumbled, "Yes, Mama," and she got off me and told me to get up so we could allow the nice man to take us into town. I glanced over at the man who was now sitting in the chair rubbing his dick and he just looked at me and smiled.

    The entire time we were in town, I was in pain from where she hit me in my back. The man kept touching me, but her focus was on spending his money and me straightening up my face. I never got a piece of the steak, but she did steal me several candy bars. She knew that I loved candy, and no matter what type of mood I was in or how I was being treated, a candy bar always made me feel better. In her own weird way, this was her way of telling me she was sorry. My mom was pitiful, and I was so ashamed of her.

My sister was growing older and more distant. She was out of the house more often, and she really did not listen to my mother. Developmentally, my sister and I were far more advanced than the average, because we learned at a young age that we had to get out there and fend for ourselves. **It became the norm to come home to a passed-out mother, dirty dishes, cold house, no food, and just plain bullshit as I then defined my life!** I think my sister secretly hated me, because she probably felt like she had warned me that we should have stayed with Grandma and Grandpa or our aunt and uncle. The social workers continued to come to school, and we always lied. But it was evident that we had a lack of attendance, and I always looked homeless when they came to the school. They began to make unannounced visits to our house, and we would sit in the house and listen to them knock on the door. I really wanted help, but I just did not know what to do except roll with the punches, because I felt as though the social workers were not going to save me, and nothing was going to change. At this point in my life, I had lost hope.

My body was beginning to develop more into a woman's body, so my mom and grandma were always accusing me of allowing boys to play with my breasts. But the truth of the matter was I afraid of boys, and even though I played with them, I would never allow one to touch me. My grandmother had told me far too many stories that had me afraid of what a man could do to me if I allowed him to have sex with me, and because I had come into contact with so many perverts, the whole concept of a man was a turnoff. However, this did not keep my mom or grandma from calling me names such as sluts and bitches. The name-calling became the norm, and it no longer affected me. My sister was never home, and it seemed that my mother did not harass my sister like she did me. I believe that my mom knew that my sister would fight her back, so I was always the target, and my sister was never there to protect me. I thought my sister was having sex, but I never asked her and she never told, but I knew that she was dating. I always felt as though she was much prettier than me, and I was always left to complete her chores. Hell, I was always lying and covering for her, but it was okay, because I was the one that created this life for us. So I felt as though I should have to pay for it, too.

More Life-Changing Events

One night, I had been really sick and was in the bed wondering why life was this way. I had been running a temperature and sweating profusely. My mom had managed to be home for a few days, because my brother was a little sick, too. One thing I knew for sure was she was not there for me; but no matter how bad she was on drugs, she always managed to be there for my brother. At this point, we had lost our trailer and were now staying with my brother's dad. It was reside there or with Grandma, and I spent my time between both homes. But one thing was for sure: I could not escape from some form of abuse regardless of what end of the spectrum I was on. So, as I was lying in the bed, I heard my mom say, "Angel, get your black ass down here." I got out of the bed in pain, wondering what the hell her ass wanted now, and I looked down the hall. She said, "Your damn brother done spit up everywhere, and I need you to come clean this shit up." I said, "But Mom, I am sick, too, and I don't feel good." "I don't give a fuck what you are, and when I tell your black ass to do something, you fucking do it. Do you fucking hear me?" She sounded like a fucking madwoman! I said, "I am coming," in my very meek and afraid voice. As I proceeded down the hall, I was crying, and I watched her and my brother sit in the bed. He had a devilish smirk on his face; I truly believe that this is why he and I do not have a sisterly-brotherly relationship today because of his treatment towards me when I was living there.

As soon as I hit the bathroom where he had spit up, I immediately cried harder. *He knew he could have spit up in the toilet*, I thought. I got on my knees, crying and trying not to cry too loud because I did not want to get the shit beat out of me. Just then, my sister walked through the door. I knew she was high, because at this point we were very familiar with what drugs were, and my sister had began smoking marijuana on a daily basis. I heard her ask, "Angel, where are you?" Sobbing, I mustered enough strength to say, "In the bathroom." She came in the room, looked at my mom and brother, and asked, "Why the hell you down there cleaning up that shit and you sick?" I said, "Because Momma told me to." She said, "Get up, Angel, and I will do it for you. Just go get back in the bed." My mom got up out of the bed and said, "Who the fuck do you think you are? You don't run a mutherfucking thing up in this house. I said she going' to clean that shit up. "Angel, you better not move and I want you to get that shit cleaned up, now." Again, I was so afraid of my mom, the only defense I had was to cry. My sister said, "Angel, get up and go get in the bed." Then, she turned to my mom and asked, "Why your fat lazy ass don't do it?" They kept arguing over me, and finally I said, "Peaches, its okay. I will clean it." My sister came to help pick me off the floor, and my mom grabbed my sister and began choking her against the wall. I got up and was just crying. My sister said, "Go upstairs," all while she was being choked. As I turned to leave, my mom grabbed my hair, and my sister pounded on her ass like I had never seen anyone pound on someone. My sister had enough of my mom abusing us, and it was evident by the way she was hitting my mom. They were fighting like men in the street. Then, my mom got the broom and started beating my sister with the broom. I couldn't do anything but beg them to stop. I was so afraid of my mom, because she was very strong. She was hitting my sister with the broom like she was not her daughter. My sister was very small compared to my mom, but she fought a good fight. I wanted to help, but I was so afraid.

My sister got away and ran into the bedroom, and I was right with her. She was hurt really bad, but she told me that she was leaving and never coming back. I begged her not to go, but she told me that she was pregnant and going to live with her boyfriend. She urged me to get help and not be afraid to tell what my mother was doing to us. Though my sister was hurt really bad—she was limping and bleeding—she mustered up enough strength to go out the window. She kissed me and told me she loved me! She told me that I had to learn how to stand up for myself and fight back. I knew nothing about fighting, and I was too afraid to try and fight. After my sister left, I cleaned up that bullshit, and my mother and brother sat in the bed as though nothing happened. The last thing my mom said to me that night was, "Don't let me see that bitch back around here, and you better not let her in this house. She wants to be grown, let her ass be grown and make a living by herself."

The next day I went to school and finally told the administration everything that happened and where I thought my sister was. They sent the police and social workers. My sister had to go to the hospital; she had suffered many bruises, but the baby was going to be okay. I was taken home by the social workers and the police. I didn't understand why only my sister was removed from the home that day, but that was the worst thing that could have ever happened. My mom and sister did not say one word to each other. I was angry that I was being left behind. How can there be enough evidence to move one child but not the other. My mom was pissed, but I swore I did not know anything. She vowed to me that if I ever tried any of the shit that my sister did, she would kill me! I believed her with my whole heart, because I knew this bitch was crazy!

I hated social workers. I believed that they created more harm than help. They took my sister and left me.

So my sister was gone, placed in a foster home, waiting to get approval to go and live with my dad, who had recently gotten out of jail and was living in an apartment with his new woman. And there I was, stuck with a crazy lady and a brother that I hated, whose dad treated him like gold and treated me like shit! And he was always fighting my momma; as much as I hated her, I hated to see them fight. They fought with pots, pans and shovels. I remember he beat my mom so bad with a shovel that she was hospitalized for several weeks. The entire time she was in the hospital, I never went to see her. I did not care if she died; secretly, I wanted her to die. During her stay in the hospital, I had to spend more time with my grandmother, and this did not make things any better. I asked about my mom periodically, but it was not out of concern I was hoping that my request would be answered and she would die! However, I never got the news that I desired to hear.

With time, I got older, stronger, and angrier. I eventually grew tired of Mom beating the shit out of me and calling me names. I was back and fourth between my grandma and her; they lived right down the street from each other. My grandma was crazy as hell, too, and I understood some of my mom's ways after getting to know my grandma more. If you look at people and their history, it will tell you a lot about them. I now truly understand the definition of generational curses and learned behavior. My grandma taught me how to steal, and I became very good at doing so. She would make me go in the store and steal food, clothes and other miscellaneous items. If I ever got caught, she would beat the living hell out of me and swear that she taught me better than that! She would always tell me to never get caught. I would later become a professional thief [thanks, Grandma]. That is how I learned to have nice things without a damn dime to my name. (It's called surviving.)

At this point in my life, I was receiving so many beatings between my grandma and mom that I became immune. I was slowly beginning to wild out, not follow any of the rules, roll my eyes, smack my lips and even take up for myself sometimes. I often thought about my sister, but I did not have much contact with her. I knew she was pregnant, but I seldom knew where she was or what she was doing. I felt as though I was just left to survive, and that is what I learned to do, survive. As usual my brother's dad always took care of him and made sure he was fed and had decent clothes on his back. Now, me on the other hand, the only time his black ass did anything for me was when he needed me to keep my brother or when he needed information about my mother's whereabouts. I hated going to school, because I was always made fun of because I wore my grandma's shoes and only had few clothes to choose from. I hated school, and I thought that kids were just plain heartless. I stayed in trouble because that was my way of crying out for help. As I grew older, my anger turned into rage. I had a crazy-ass cousin who went around shooting me in the ass with a pellet gun and would laugh the most evil laugh in the world. All my aunts and uncles were crack heads, so there was no seeking shelter from them, because they were crazy as hell. ***This family was a true example of generational curses***.

Eventually, I began getting curious about sex and exploring my body even more. Hell, if I was getting my ass kicked for my boobs growing and beginning my menses, I felt like, what is the hype about? And if all the stories that my grandmother told me were true, then why is everyone having sex? I wanted to find out. Well, my cousin and I we were really close in age so we started fooling around. We were both curious at this point in our life. I was sucking his dick, or at least I thought I was, and he was licking my pussy. (Thinking back, it makes my stomach turn to think that I was doing those types of things, but it just goes to show you what type of dysfunctional life that I had.) We were always scared to actually put the dick in the pussy, and I never got off on the other nasty stuff that we did, so eventually we stopped fooling around. I was still curious, but not enough to actually have sex. I knew messing with my cousin was not right, because it always felt nasty. But back then, it was something for us to do, because living in the county you had to be very creative when finding fun and trying to escape the madness.

He Stole the Last Piece of Childhood

I remember my uncle would always say little nasty things to me, but I never took him seriously. But his comments were very inappropriate, and they made me uncomfortable, especially with him being my uncle. I tried to tell my mom, but she would just blow it off and make it appear that I was just telling lies and that my uncle would never say those things to me. One day, she said, "If I hear you talk like that again, I will beat the shit out of your hot ass." I wanted to hit her right in the mouth when she said that, but instead, I just looked at her and thought, *if looks could kill, she would be dead today.* I remember her grabbing my shirt, pulling me close to her, and saying, "Your ass is nothing but trouble for me." I thought, *I wish she would beat me to death so that I no longer had to give her any more trouble.*

One day when she was on one of her drug escapades, my uncle was at the house with me, and he was talking his normal crazy talk. "You know that it is time for you to get that pussy loose and learn how to handle some dick. You can't keep running from it; that is the way that you going to get a man to take care of you. Now you need to let your uncle Willie put a little bit of this dick in you. I am not going to put it all in at one time. I will make sure that I take it nice and slow, just a little, so I can get it ready for your husband." I said, "Shut up, Uncle Willie. If I did want to give it up, it would not be to your ugly ass." I proceeded to lay on the sofa, praying that he would leave me alone and just leave. He followed me over to the sofa and began rubbing on my body. At this point, I felt so violated but confused at what to do, because I knew that I could not overpower him. So many thoughts were going through my head, but the only thing that I could do was just lie down and pray that he would stop. He slowly pulled down my pants and began playing with my pussy. I begged him to stop, but the strangest and saddest thing is that even though I wanted him to stop, I liked the way that he was making me feel. He started rubbing his dick on me and then put my hand on his dick. It excited me, and I never felt that before. He whispered, "Just a little. I won't hurt you." He put it on my clit, and as he started to put it in, I began to cry and reminding him that I was his niece. He told me to shut up and that he would not hurt me. But that was not true. It hurt me really bad, and I cried the entire time. When it was over, he sent me to clean up and told me that if I ever spoke one word that he would kill me. He also made sure he let me know that he was not done. He told me that each time he was going to put a little more in me each time until I could take it all. He said this way; my husband would never leave me, because I would be able to handle a big dick.

The most sick part to this point in my life was that I started enjoying having sex with my own grown-ass uncle and was sneaking to him nightly, even if we did not do anything but hump. I hated him, but I began to love the way that he made me feel. He would be outside hanging clothes on the line, and I would go outside so that I could watch him masturbate. This went on for a very long time, until my uncle finally got a girlfriend and moved away. After that, I really thought differently of myself. I felt as though I was grown and like I was the shit, and no one could tell me what to do! I even walked differently and my body began to shape quickly. My grandmother always accused me of fucking boys in the neighborhood, but she never knew it was her son that was fucking and sucking on my boobs. One day my mom had come home from another one of her long escapades and was talking shit to me about the house not being clean. I was not trying to hear it, and I let her ass know because I had enough of her and I no longer viewed her as my mother. In my eyes, she was another bitch in the streets and did not warrant my respect. I had been through so much pain in my life that her beatings no longer bothered me. They would hurt for the moment, but after it was over, I always knew that I would be okay. This night as she came towards me I did not flinch; she beat the shit out of me. I think she beat me so bad this time because she saw in my eyes the desire to fight back. The entire time she was punching me she kept telling me she would kill me if I thought about hitting her. I believe she hit harder because she knew that I had developed tough skin, ever time she knocked me down I got back up as though I was asking for more.

Whenever she hit me in a place that really hurt I would envision the first night that my uncle stole all my innocence and I would become numb to pain. That night after she grew tired and I cleaned up the house I ran away! I had nowhere to go, so the first night I climbed up in a tree in the woods and stayed there until the following day. This was very scary and I was very hungry, but as afraid as I was being in the woods all alone, I was more afraid of what she would do to me if she found me. The next day, I went to my aunt's house and hid out there until she got tired of me and told me that I had to go home. She was an addict, too, and she was cool if she was high, because then she was happy and did not care about anything. But the moment that she came down from that high, she would start tripping and want to put everyone out of the house, including her own children. I begged her not to send me away. I said, "My mom is going to kill me." My aunt laughed and said, "Your momma is not going to kill you," and I said, "You don't understand. She hates me." I told my cousin to go to school and tell the principal so they could contact social services. I truly believed that she was going to kill me when she found me. After all, I had been gone for several days and was not available to babysit my brother or to entertain her men. I had not been home in three days. I knew that the school had been calling, and she did not like for me to bring her any heat! My cousin promised that he would report it as soon as he got to school. Well, that day my mom came to my aunt's house and said, "I know that bitch is here." My aunt tried to lie, but by that time, my mom was looking in all the closets and getting closer to me. I was hiding in the bedroom closet and decided to come out before she found me. I tried to apologize, but before I could say anything, she punched me right in my lip, knocking me to the floor. She hit me several times, back to back, and I was balled up in a knot. But she never stopped hitting me, even though I cried out for her to stop.

Fist after fist she beat the living shit, and even though my aunt begged her to stop, she never intervened; she never pulled her off me. My momma beat me all the way to the car. My entire body was aching, and every step that I took, she would either hit me or kick me. When we got home, she beat me more and told me, "Now, you little bitch, you going to school tomorrow, and I don't care what you tell them white motherfuckers. I don't want your black ass anyway. I hope they come and take you, just like they took your sister." I remember she stepped on my hand when I was sitting on the steps; she broke my whole nail on my pointer finger. I vowed not to look at her, because I felt I would receive another blow to the face. As angry as I was and as much as I wanted to fight back I was so afraid of her. I thought she was the craziest bitch alive. *(Who would ever think that I would inherit some of those traits?)* The next day, I went to school, and my cousin had already reported to the principal that my mother was abusing me. I was asked by my teacher to go to the office, and there I met another CPS worker. This time, I begged her not to return me to my home. I showed her the bruises and told her that my mom was going to kill me. They took several pictures and she assured me that I would be safe and that I would not be returning home, but she had to speak with my mother. I told her she would need to bring the police, because she would kill her. I told her that my mom was not afraid of anyone! Well surely, she took to heart what I said, because the police escorted her to our house, and I rode with the worker in the car. My mom met her at the door, eyes looking big and mad as hell. She said no one was coming into her house, and she did not care who it was. Ms. Marsha attempted to ask her for my belongings and explain to her that I was not going to be returning home. My mom proudly said, "Well, she came with nothing, and she will leave with nothing." I sat in the backseat of that car, crying my eyes out, and she watched me the whole time. It was at that moment that I thought, *my own mother hates me*. So many thoughts went through my mind, but I will never forget the look in her eyes that day.

 I truly believe that if she could have choked me while I was in that car, she would have choked me until I died! As we drove away, I asked Ms. Marsha where I was going, and she told me that I was going to live with my dad for a while. She explained to me that he had an apartment with his girlfriend and that they were doing really well and my sister was already with him. This was odd, but I was happy because I always wanted to live with my dad, and it was going to be nice to be back with my sister. I was always dreaming of my dad rescuing me, so this felt like it was a dream. I was finally rescued, and a little bit of my physical and emotional pain slowly subsided. It would be years before I would see my mom again! A deep place in my heart was praying that my dad would not turn into a monster like my mom.

More Dysfunction

I remember when I arrived at my dad's, I felt so odd. I knew him, but I did not know him. His girlfriend appeared to be phony, and my spirit did not like something about her. It would not be long before I learned that my dad was an alcoholic and a drug addict himself. It appeared that I was moved from one crazy house to the next. This house was full of name-calling and located in the projects, and we were never supervised. My bed consisted of several blankets on the floor, and food was limited. I would soon learn that my so-called stepmom was the wicked witch from the east! She would lock up food from my sister and me and only feed us what she wanted us to eat. She was so evil, and I hated her. My dad saw no wrong in her, but I believe that was because he could not do any better for himself. I soon encountered more men who would always try to sneak around a corner and rub on me, and my dad would be too drunk to realize what was going on. I was beginning to think that something was wrong with me. Why did I always attract men who wanted to hurt me sexually? I never did anything to bring this type of attention to me, and I sure did not feel pretty. I had no decent clothes, and my hair was always knotty.

Living in the projects introduced me to a whole different set of people. I got in with the wrong crowd, because I was trying to find myself. My sister was never at home, and when I did see her, she was always high. She never talked about what happened with the baby and I never asked. One day I told her to teach me how to smoke. I will never forget the first time I smoked a Newport cigarette. My sister, along with all the other fat-ass girls in the neighborhood, laughed at me. She said, "Nigga, you not inhaling." So I said, "Well, teach me." I choked the first time that I actually inhaled. I regret ever learning how to smoke, because I always thought they were nasty. But whenever I was stressed out, angry, depressed, or hungry, a cigarette always did the trick of making me feel better.

As time progressed, I became more and more enmeshed in the streets. The streets became my home away from home. The people in the hood loved me far more than the home life. I was always down to do whatever. If someone told me to do something, I would do it, because I wanted to always be down and to build a reputation for myself. I will never forget standing outside of a 7-11, and I was told that if I wanted to show that I was down with the Centerville clique, I would have to prove it by hitting an innocent person in the head. So, the moment I saw a white girl walk out of the store, I took my soda and bust her right in the head, and I would not stop hitting her. She tried to run and I ran after her, spitting on her and pulling out her hair. I watched the white girl cry and beg me to stop, and when I finally did, she asked me why did I do this and what did she do? I had no answer, and even though a secret part of me wanted to apologize, share the tears with her, and tell her that I never meant to do it, there was an evil side to me that just did not care because of all the mean things that had been done to me. So the only thing that I could say was, "Because bitch, you deserved it. Now get the fuck out of here before I beat your ass again!" That day, I was considered to be the shit in the hood, and now I had respect! We all left the store, running before the cops came.

It was not long before I learned about "lack of supervision." This was what was told to me when I was taken from my dad. I was always in trouble by now and didn't give a damn about anything. I had managed to hold onto my virginity, but I was smoking, skipping school, going to court, and kicking ass! After my first fight at the store, it felt good to be able to get my anger out by using someone as a punching bag. I had caught two assault and battery charges in less than six months of living with my dad. No one seemed to notice me unless I was in trouble. My dad was a stone-cold alcoholic and a drug addict. My dad did not physically abuse me, but the neglect was ever so present, I rarely saw my sister, and my so called step-mom was just evil and the only time she smiled was when she needed a favor.

So, eventually, along came another social worker and a probation officer who tried to dictate to me whom I could see and gave me a list of rules that I was surely not about to follow. I felt as though that I was in charge, and no one was going to tell me how to run my life. It was 1993 when I met my first probation officer; I was eleven years old. The first charge that led me to her was assault and battery. She did not like my attitude, and I did not like her attitude. I would later find out that she was the one who filed a complaint against my dad. I always wondered how she knew everything: it was because she was on her game and very much involved in my well-being. She was the type of probation officer who went beyond the call of duty and definitely outside her nine to five. This woman would come to the hood and make it known that she was there. I felt as though she was always harassing me and wanting to drug test me, knowing that I was going to be dirty. I did not understand that then, but I certainly do thank her now! She held me accountable for every action, and even though I tried to be grown, she saw the child in me that desired to be a child, that desired some structure and more importantly desired to be loved.

Crazy crack cocaine was being sold out of our house by everyone who lived there, and we had a lot of people living in our home. It was called "running out the crack house." My probation officer was always asking me about the reports of drugs being sold and used in my home, and I would just look at her as though I had no clue as to what she was talking about. She eventually placed me on house arrest, which I thought was for the birds. This form of house arrest consisted of people calling to check on me and me having to call them. If I was not home or did not report on time, I would receive a violation. *Whatever* is what I thought. I was too deep in the streets, and so was everyone else who lived in my home. But I tell you one thing: we could put on a show whenever those "white folks" would come to our house. We referred to anyone as a "white folk" if they were trying to get into our business, regardless of whether they were white or black. However, I believe that Ms. Miller (my probation officer) and my other counselor saw through our line of bullshit! It was not long before I was violated for violation of house arrest and got my first air of detention. I vowed to never go back. It was definitely not a place for me. There were people telling me what to do, what to eat, how long to shower, and what time to turn off my lights. While we were showering, the counselors use to say to us in detention "fruit, cock tail": that was the time that we were permitted to shower. That meant wash your ass, your underarms, and get out of the shower! I hated detention, and I hated having to shower with several other girls and having total strangers see my body.

After being released, I was placed back in the home with my dad, but it was not long before I was removed and placed with my first foster parent. The reasoning that was given to me for my removal was there was a lack of supervision. I was vexed, because even though my dad was never home and I barely had food to eat, it was still home, and I did not want to leave he did not beat me and I was able to take care of myself! I don't remember much about my first foster mom except for the fact that I did not like her. I had begged my grandfather to take me, because I did not like living with her. She was mean and sneaky. I felt as though she was always putting on a show to try and impress my social worker. But behind closed doors, she did not give a damn about me. Eventually, my grandfather agreed to have me come and live with him, but he had many stipulations, but I would have said yes to anything to get out of my current living situation. My social worker allowed this to take place, and, of course, there was a long list of rules, which I did not follow.

I hated staying with my granddad and my aunt Quince; she was just as crazy as my grandma! I finally understood why my grandma hated her. My grandma had seven kids by my grandpa, and now her own sister was living with him and sleeping with him every day. Talk about dysfunction! Quince was crazy and was known to be verbally abusive, but she knew I was crazy, too, so she never tried any of her bullshit with me. I later found out that she did not want me living there, but they both agreed, because money came along with my stay. My granddad was poor, and his house looked as though poor people stayed in. I was always made to cut wood which is how we heated the house, and we had to heat the water on the stove to take a wash up. I was so embarrassed, but being embarrassed eventually became something that I was immune to. I was always telling lies to my granddad, and I always thought I was getting over and that he was the biggest fool! Granddad had a demeanor that required respect, and I never disrespected him other than with my lies. I was afraid of him, because I believed in my heart that he was the Incredible Hulk!

One day I got suspended from school, and my granddad had to come pick me up. We were about five minutes from the school, and he pulled over on the road and told me to get out. I looked at him with a puzzled look on my face, and he said that I had to walk home as part of my punishment. I was pissed, because home was about an hour walking distance. Then he said that when I got home, I was not to touch the telephone. I got out of the car and he pulled away. So I walked home. I knew that I no longer wanted to live with my granddad, so when I finally reached to the house, I got right on the phone to plan my escape. As time progressed, I found out that my grandfather was calling social services and my probation officer, telling them everything that I was doing. It was not long before I was back in the courts for violation of probation. This time, I was placed on electronic monitoring, which meant I had to wear this ugly black beeper around my leg that would send a signal every time I left home or school. They had me on lock, monitoring my every move. I was pissed. I also received another outreach worker, who was in charge of monitoring my house arrest and conducting impromptu visits. She was white, but there was something that I liked about this woman. I would soon learn that it was her spirit and that she actually cared about me! It was not just a paycheck for her. This white lady went out of her way for me, all the while holding me accountable. I can remember when I told her that we did not have any food, and she showed up with several bags of groceries. Our relationship was so close that she allowed me to come to her home, shower, and meet her children, who were just as wonderful and sweet as she was. Ms. Spain was the person who introduced me to coffee. She taught me how to make the best coffee. I secretly wished that I could go and live with her, but she never asked me to come, so I assumed she never wanted me.

Though many services attempted to assist with stabilizing me, I was too far gone, too angry and deep in the streets. It was not long before I was removed from my granddads and placed in detention for violation of house arrest. It was funny, but sometimes the only time I really saw my sister was while in detention. Our relationship was so strange, my sister had a baby and I barely knew her. I think between her being born and turning three, I maybe saw her two times. After my third trip to detention, I would soon learn about "upstate." This is what they consider the juvenile version of penitentiary. Being committed upstate introduced me too far more than what I had gotten myself involved with on the streets. I was locked up with girls who had killed their parents and had been sentenced to juvenile life as young as thirteen years old. Until this point, I never thought that I would meet someone else who hated there parents so much that they not only wanted to kill them but went through with the act of killing them.

Being committed upstate, I had to learn how to get tough skin. I was no longer just living in the 757. I now had to interact with girls from Richmond and throughout the state of Virginia. Going upstate is where I first learned about drug trafficking and how much money that I could make. I also learned about lesbianism and the reason why most females got "turned out." My first trip upstate was fairly short, but I vowed never to return. I hated the food, and I hated having to be shackled to another inmate every time we were transported somewhere, including the mess hall.

After my release, I was placed in a therapeutic foster home, whatever that meant. I remember that I was told that the lady would be coming to visit me while I was upstate. The day that she was due to come, I was nervous because I wanted her to like me, and I wanted to like her. I was afraid that she would think that I was ugly. My hair was a mess, because being upstate, there was no such thing as perms and hairdos. I walked into the visitation room, and there sat a beautiful black woman, who looked evil as hell. Next to her was my white social worker, who I could not stand. I always felt as though she put on this big front, as though she was such a caring person who wanted the best for the kids on her caseload. But deep down inside, I thought she was a witch and that she hated me and wanted me to spend the rest of my life locked up so that her life would be much easier not having to deal with me or find me homes. Anyway, as she began to introduce me to my prospective foster parent, I immediately cut her off and said as rudely as I could, "What you want me for?" I looked this lady right in her eyes. I asked, "Do you know my history, did they tell you that I was crazy?" She continued to look at me and finally asked, "Are you done?" I then looked at my social worker and asked, sarcastically, "Am I done?" That's when my social worker asked, "Angel, do you want to get out of here?" And naturally, me being the smart ass that I was, I replied, "If your fat ass was in here, would you want to get out? Hell yes, I want to leave!" Ms. Pee (the foster lady) began talking to me about my likes and dislikes. She talked with me about her son and her husband. My final question was, "When do I leave?" My social worker said that I would be discharged within a week and that I would have strict guidelines of parole to abide by. She made sure that she reminded me that if I messed up, I would be right back upstate. I thought, *Shit, I am never coming back to this hellhole.*

Losing My Virginity and My Mind in My New Foster Home

It amazes me that we foster children can be abused, neglected, and downright treated like shit by our biological parents, but we still manage to love them and always want to return home no matter what conditions we may return home to. While I was upstate, my dad came to visit me one time, and I was so happy; he could always make me laugh. Out of the many trips that I made to detention, that was the only visit I ever received from my dad or anyone else. And even that visit was full of lies about how he was working hard to be able to get me back home. That Nigga wasn't working on anything but getting high and drunk every day. But he was my dad, and I loved him. As for my mom, I never heard from her, and I really did not care. I never tried to call her, and I believe that as each day passed, I grew more and more hate for her.

When I got to my new foster-home placement, my foster mother showed me my room, and my mattress was on the floor. I didn't care, because anything was better than being upstate, and her house was clean. Hell, I was so use to sleeping on the floor that having a mattress made me feel as though I was living large and privileged. But in the back of my mind, I thought, *how in the hell can a foster parent only have a mattress for a foster child to sleep on.* She promised me that I would have a bed soon. I also met my two new foster brothers. One was her biological son, whom I loved immediately, and the other was this crazy-ass foster child, and I would soon kick his ass. Mr. Pee was never home; he always had to work or was sleeping. He was very humble and never said much. Mrs. Pee took me to get my hair done, and I felt like a princess. I had never been to a hair salon before. That lady put a perm in my hair that made me think I was an Indian. Next, I had to be enrolled in school. I was enrolled in alternative school that was full of bad-ass kids just like me. I asked my foster mom what I should call her. I did not want the other students to know that I was in foster care. I don't think that we ever really came to an agreement, so I tried to never call her, because I was not comfortable calling her anything. We never really bonded. I was always in trouble at school, and I think I got on her nerves, because she was always having to transport me somewhere or pick me up from school, all while dealing with the other foster child and her biological son.

Eventually I hooked up with an old friend, and we began spending a lot of time together. I really don't think my foster mom cared, because it kept me from the house. He was always trying to get in my panties, and I was afraid, but everyone was talking about sex. I was looking for love in all the wrong places, and I thought I had found it in him. I will never forget the day when I finally gave in. Aaron had promised to love me always and to take me away from all this madness. The first time it hurt like hell, and it was very uncomfortable. I thought that I would enjoy it, but a big part of my virginity had already been stolen when I was a little girl. To my surprise, after when we were done, Aaron looked at me and said, "You are not a virgin." I began crying and said, "Yes I

Wounded, But Not Broken

am!" He said, "If you were a virgin, you would be bleeding." I had no words for him, and I felt totally violated and disrespected. After Aaron saw how much he hurt me, he was very apologetic, but I still think he did not believe me, and slowly our relationship began to dwindle. I did not know anything about love, and I was so bitter I did not know how to express myself. I don't think I ever really loved Aaron, and I had no business having sex. It was a long time before I ever did it again. I found out early in the game if you were giving up the pussy then the boys were plenty, but they drifted away quickly as soon as they found out that you were not going to be screwing them. I think God every day that despite what had happened to me, I did not become another promiscuous victim. It took a long time for anyone to be able to have sex with me, and it took even longer for me to really experience an orgasm and understand the true art of making love.

By this time, I was sick of being away from my so-called family. I was sick of these "white people" telling me what to do and even more sick of the rules of parole. I kept trying to get a visit with my dad, and every time they would tell me he was not doing what he was suppose to do. Then I would call him, and he would sell me a bunch of lies that I wanted to believe. One day I was arguing with the other foster child, and he was saying some really cruel things. I was on the phone with my dad, and he came and snatched the phone out of the hook. I went and told Ms. Pee, who was right in the kitchen at the time, and she gave him a little mild reprimand. I got very angry and asked, "That's all you going to say?" Secretly, I believe she wanted me to whip his ass! So I gave her what she wanted. I went into the living room and asked him why he hung up on my dad? He said, "He don't want your dumb' ass anyway." I said, "And your momma doesn't want your retarded, stuttering ass." He was a lot bigger than I, so the moment I saw him get his ass off that sofa, I charged him like a bull and began laying blows straight to his head. I had him pinned down on the floor, and Ms. Pee was yelling for us to stop before we woke Christopher (her son). So, as I attempted to get off him, I rubbed his head in the carpet some more. But as I was getting up, he hit me in the eye. He hit me so hard water immediately starting running out my eye, and I could not see. He took off, running outside. I went to the kitchen and grabbed a butcher knife; I was going to kill him. Ms. Pee begged me to stop, and by this time, she was calling the cops and had locked the bolt lock from inside so that I could not go out the door. I begged her not to call the cops, but she said she had to. I knew that I had to leave, so I went out the window. I never saw any of them again.

I stayed on the run for a long time. One thing that I learned about the streets and people, they are both heartless. No one wants you to live for free, eat for free, or run up there water bill for free. The streets taught me about money, sex, drugs, and survival. By this time, I was still young, but full figured. I never had much of an ass, but my boobs said, "Damn!" I was smoking and drinking like crazy and surviving by whatever means necessary. I remember being so drunk one time that I peed on this guy's living room floor. I was so drunk I could not do anything but laugh. It was not long before he had me in his car, with the windows up and the doors locked. He told me how I was a stupid bitch, peeing on his momma's floor. I remember him telling me he was going to fuck me real good. I was drunk, but I knew I was about to be raped. I tried to tell him to stop, but he kept sucking me everywhere; I felt like he was biting me. I kept my hand in front of my pussy, but he was much stronger than I, and I was very drunk. I prayed that my girlfriend would come to the car and rescue me, and the Lord again heard my cry and brought her and everyone else outside. I was kicking the window, and she begged him to stop or she was going to bust the windows and call the police! He finally stopped, after sucking me real good on my face for several minutes. He opened the door and kicked me out of the car. My girl picked me up while everyone else was just looking. She got me into the car, and we drove home. The next day, my pussy was very sore from where he kept trying to put all his fingers in me, and my body felt as though I had been stampeded on by a herd of elephants. This guy had scarred me with hickeys all over my face, neck, and shoulders. I began to cry and asked my girl if he had raped me. She said, "Almost." I vowed to never drink again. I was fucked up and didn't know what to do. My girl and I never really talked about what happened. I couldn't blame her, because we were all drinking. Several days later, this guy had the nerve to call me as though everything was cool and nothing ever happened. I told him if I ever saw him again, I would kill him. It's funny because I was so young, but I meant every word! I would soon learn that getting drunk was not the thing to do and that it leads to problems. But this was only the first; it should have been the last, but it was not!

Around this same time, I was running with one of the biggest drug dealers, (Carlos). We started out as really good friends. To me, he was like the father and mother that I longed to have. Friends eventually turned into lovers, and lovers eventually turned into him whipping my ass.

Let me define "whipping my ass." This guy would kick me, stomp me, hit me in my face in a crowd, beat me in my face with a curtain rod, and leave several bruises on my face. One day he stomped me in my head so hard that his Timberland footprint was left on the right side of my face. These beatings where frequent and I was only about thirteen or fourteen years old, but life for me was real!

I knew that I could not allow him to see me with those hickeys on my neck. He would have sworn that I was out sleeping around. So I had to find a place to stay where I would be able to duck him for at least a week, until those awful hickeys went away. Carlos was crazy, and I honestly felt as though he was capable of killing me. I can honestly say that I was afraid of him. During this time, I stayed with different people, and each one of them treated me differently. But none of them ever made me feel comfortable, clean, or loved.

The streets taught me how to feed myself with little to no money. I would go to Burger King and get me a Whopper after scraping up some change. I would eat half of the Whopper, put a piece of my hair in the Whopper, and go back up there and piss a bitch until I got another full meal. My belly would be full for the day. During this time of hiding from Carlos and the police, I was getting sick of living place to place and was ready for another visit to detention. In detention, I always knew I was safe, other than an occasional fight. In detention, we had three meals and a snack and a hot shower that was mandatory.

One night I was out with one of my fake-ass girlfriends at this house where many dope boys ran. We were in the house chilling, getting high as hell, and laughing our asses off when Carlos entered. I could have shit in my pants I was so nervous, but I was trying to be cool about everything. He came up to me and planted a kiss right on my cheek. He then whispered in my ear, "You have been hiding from me?" I attempted to say no, but before I could, he had yanked me off the sofa and started shoving me outside. My girlfriend asked Carlos to please leave me alone, but she was quickly shut up by the other nigga's in the house. It did not take much for her to fall back and not try to help me anymore. He got me outside and pulled out his gun. He told me that I played too many games, and he was going to show me how much he loved me. I couldn't say anything, because I did not know what to say. He told me to talk, and I knew that he meant every word. The moment I opened my mouth, he shot the gun by my foot. I immediately started crying. Everyone came running outside, like, "Nigga, you crazy." My girl, Nikki, pleaded with him not to hurt me. He asked every last guy out there if they were fucking me. Everyone looked at Carlos as though he was crazy, and Crook finally spoke up and said, "Man, nobody fucking your girl!" I was crying hysterically, and before I knew it, he was shooting the gun again. This time, he shoved me off the porch and down a flight of five stairs. I landed right in the mud. He immediately said, "Get your dumb ass up and get in the car." I said, "I do not want to go with you," and he shot one more time and then promised that he would not miss again. I got in the car, sobbing and embarrassed. Nikki sat in the front seat with Reese, and Carlos sat in the backseat with me. He told me that he loved me and that was why he did those things. He put the gun to my head and told me that I could never leave him. We got to the hotel, and he made me take a shower. I lay on the sofa, sobbing, and he came and raped me. *Now, when I say rape in this context, I mean mentally and emotionally. I did not want to sleep with this man at all, but mentally I have been getting raped all my life, and eventually being raped physically began to feel good. But it was killing me emotionally and mentally.*

The next day, when it was time to check out of the room, I felt unclean. Carlos always wanted to beat on me if he thought that I was sleeping around, but I knew that he was sleeping with almost all the girls in the hood. Carlos took me to my uncle's house, dropped me off, and told me he would see me later I knew that he was going to see another one of his girls, but I did not care. I thought to myself as he drove off, *you won't ever see me again!* As soon as he dropped me off, I went in, took a shower, and listened to my uncle talk shit about the cops looking for me and me making his house hot. I slept all day and then was up looking for something to smoke. I caught a ride down to the hood, hooked up with some of my peeps, and got high as hell. I was hungry and trying very hard not to see Carlos. I remember walking down the street, feeling lonely and sad and thinking that life at some point had to get better. I wondered what my dad was doing and if he even cared that his daughter was on the run. I wondered where my sister was, and I had a rage shoot up in my body when I started thinking about my mother. I hated that woman so much, and I blamed everything on her! My life was a living hell, and I never understood how a mother could be in a world and not give a shit about her children. As I walked, deep into thought and with tears flowing down my face, I saw a cop. I immediately started to run, but instead I stopped, stood there, and flagged him down. It was time to go home to my familiar place that gave me a safety net, the place called detention.

The police officer pulled over, and I gave him all my information. I told him I was on parole and was currently on the run. He took no time placing me in handcuffs, but this time I did not bother to put up a fight, it was my pleasure. I had to sit in intake for a long time, waiting to be arraigned. I was allowed to speak to my parole officer, and, of course, she told me that she was disappointed, but happy that I decided to turn myself in. This time I found out that I was really being shipped far away. They were sending me to Christiansburg. I had never heard of the place, but I was in for a rude awakening. Christiansburg was in red neck city, and this detention was full of white staff, which was not the norm for me. Being placed in this detention center was by far my worst experience (literally). I counted the walls at least a thousand times. All the boys in this detention center were weird. I was the only black girl, but there were some really cool white girls. The funny thing is that I always hear people talk about the number of black adolescents who are detained, but I promise you, in my many detention stays, the whites always had us outnumbered.

One day we were sitting at the mess hall, and I was talking plenty of shit to this guy with very large ears. Before I knew it he was up out of his seat and had hit me in my head. I immediately got up and went to retaliate, but the lazy staff had finally gotten him restrained. I was rushed to the hospital and received six stitches in my forehead and a black eye—all with one hit! I was hurt badly, and when I got back to the detention center, I received indefinite lockdown. I was pissed and did not understand why I had to be locked down. I was told that I instigated the fight. I was in pain, but I went the hell off, and everything was taken out of my room because I promised to kill myself. I stayed locked down in the room so long I literally made myself sick. I believe that if I had something to kill myself with, I would have done it. While on lockdown, a new admission came in who apparently knew the boy that I had the altercation with. She came to my door one time and told me to watch my back, because she was going to kick my ass. I never responded, but I thought, "Bitch, I will kill you!" I sat back, laughing like I was a crazy person. That night, when staff came so that I could get a shower, I remember her still talking shit! The next thing I knew, she was coming out for her shower. I made sure staff did not see me, and I took my soap and wrapped it in a towel. I knew who she was, because she was the only other black inmate, and she had come to my little window talking shit on several occasions. As soon as she entered the bathroom, the staff told me that time was up, and it was time for me to get out of the shower. I immediately came out swinging. I did not give her a chance to say one word. I beat the shit out of her, and it took a lot of manpower to get me off her! I went back to my hole, laughing the whole way. "I bet you won't talk shit no more," was the last thing that I said to her.

The next day, I got a phone call from my probation officer, and she told me that I would be released and placed with my dad on a temporary basis. I was elated. I asked her how, and she said that after he found out that I had got hurt, he talked with my social worker and began taking several classes that he needed in order to have me returned home. *Damn, the old man actually cared*, I thought. My probation officer apologized for what happened to me and said she never meant for me to be in an unsafe place where people would allow that to happen. She told me staff should have never allowed him to get that close to me, and she was disappointed in the facility. She also inquired about the fight that I had been in with the young lady. I explained to her that she was threatening me and that I had to get her before she got me. One thing that I can say about my probation officer: I could always be honest with her. I hated her, but I loved her, too. I stayed in my room and served those remaining ten days waiting for and anticipating my release. When I was finally discharged, I told all the staff I did not like to kiss my ass.

Back at Home with My Dad

Seeing those sheriffs pick me up was wonderful. I had become very close with Deputy Cookie. She was the sweetest sheriff you ever wanted to meet. She loved me, and she has always looked out for me on every transport. She also told me that I was beautiful and gifted and there was more to me than getting in trouble. I never disrespected Ms. Cookie. When I got back in front of the judge, I was very polite, and he told me he did not want to see me back in his courtroom. He also spoke with my dad, whom I was so happy to see. He told him that he had been given a second chance and that he needed to provide me with supervision and support. He also reminded my dad of all the classes that he needed to continue in order to regain my custody. I soon found out that being with my dad was only on a trial basis, and even though I was living with him, social services still had my custody, and I still had to have them all in my business. My probation officer also made sure that she included that I be court ordered to attend school daily, submit to random drug testing, and have a strict curfew of 8:00 every night. I would have agreed to anything to be able to get out of that courthouse. My dad told me that he was sorry I got hit, but then he made a joke and asked, "Did you get any licks in?" I laughed and said, "No, but I surely tried!" As soon as I got home, I saw my sister who now also had a son. I was happy to see her, but she acted as though we were living together all of our lives and that she saw me everyday. She was not happy to see me. It appeared that my sister and I just had a strained relationship. My dad's home was a two-bedroom apartment, and it was junky as hell, but I did not care. My fake step mom greeted me as usual, and I greeted her with my phony attitude and acted as though I was happy to see her. I really did not care; I was just happy to be around family. It was not long before my dad told me that Carlos had been around several times, looking for me. I begged him not to tell him that I was home. My dad said that he already knew that I was coming home today. I told my dad that I did not want to see Carlos. My dad said, "Well, he is coming by, and he has been giving us money to give to you and to help out." I was pissed Carlos had already started manipulating my dad. I told my dad about all the mean things and brutal beatings that Carlos had done to me, and my dad's only response was that I had to be doing something to make him want to beat on me.

I looked at my dad as though he was crazy to say that to his daughter, but then I remembered whom I was talking to, so and I decided not to fight that battle. So, to prevent an argument, I quickly changed the subject and told my dad that my stomach had been hurting me really bad since I went to detention. My dad took me to the hospital, and there I found out that I had Chlamydia. I cried my eyes out. I knew that Carlos had given it to me. I was so ashamed when they told me in front of my dad. They told me that Chlamydia sometimes lays dormant, and it may take several weeks before symptoms begin. They were going to treat me immediately, because it could cause sterilization. I was given some pills that I had to take for seven days to assure that it was all gone. I begged my dad not to say anything, and he promised me that he would not. The first thing the next day, I heard a knock at the door, and it was Carlos. I looked him dead in the face and asked him to please leave me alone. I told him what he had given me, and he asked, "Did you get me some pills, too?" Everything was a joke to him. He said he was sorry and that things happen. He told me to get dressed, because we were going to get my hair done and he was taking me shopping. He knew just what to say! He took me out, bought me some clothes, got my hair done, and even respected me when I told him I did not want to have sex. We stayed together that night and then he took me home in the morning, because I had to be enrolled in school.

Being back in public school felt strange and I did not like it at all. School created a lot of problems for me. I spent more time harassing the teachers and other students than I did learning. It was not long before I was in trouble for skipping school and fighting. I just had an "I don't care" attitude. I was happy to be back with my dad, but I had a gut feeling that it was not going to be long before I was moved again. My dad was still doing his thing, and so was I. I remember one day going outside and walking to the corner store. I ran into Carlos, and he immediately told me to get into the car. I told him that I was not going with him and asked him to please leave me alone and respect my wishes. He went onto to tell me that I was nothing without him. I continued to walk off; because I knew that he was capable of doing anything. He got out of the car and poured a forty-ounce bottle of beer onto me. He laughed and told me to go clean up and that I had thirty minutes to get home, and I was to be ready when he came to pick me up. I cried and reminded him of my curfew. He said that he knew my dad would cover for me. He kissed me and drove off. I went into the house, crying, and I told my dad what had happened. He told me that he was going to take care of it right away. I later found out that my dad went and looked for Carlos, but once he got hooked up with some free crack, he left alone the whole situation about the beer being thrown on me. So that night

I went with Carlos. That was another bad decision. I never returned home, because I knew that I would be violated. While I was on the run this time, I caught a weed charge and was caught in an abandoned building after several guys had shot at us repeatedly. We were too afraid to try and leave the scene, because we did not know if someone would be outside waiting for us. After the police arrived, I tried to lie about my name and age, but that did not work. Carlos even tried to get me out by saying that he was my uncle, but it did not work. Eventually, the officer told me that he would file additional charges against me for giving false information, so I told him my real name. They transported me straight to Newport News Detention. This time, I had to do several weeks, and I was told that my father was not able to provide the supervision and parenting that I needed, so I would be placed back in a foster home. They tried to soften things by telling me that I would be close to my family, but that did not make me feel better. At this point in my life, I did not care about anything, and everyone I encountered was a liar; I no longer trusted anyone. My probation officer made sure she told me that I was not to have any contact with Carlos. I really did not care, because I was tired of him whipping my ass. This time, I was placed in a foster home that was located in downtown Newport News.

More Foster Home's

This foster mom was single and lived by herself in a very old home. She was strange, and she did not talk much. She also lived in the hood. This is the neighborhood where I would first develop my fear of cats. Every time I went outside, I would see big nasty cats and drunks on the corner, always trying to bum a dollar. There was no change in my school behavior; I continued to fight and cause problems that required my foster mom to come to the school. I called my social worker almost every day requesting to be moved, and the majority of the time, she would never return my phone call. I felt as though if I continued to give this woman hell, she would eventually say I had to get out of her house. I was always sad and depressed, and I told my social worker that I was going to commit suicide. The next thing I knew, they had me in front of a psychiatrist, and she asked me several questions and showed me several different pictures of different figures. I was a little vexed and asked this lady what was I suppose to see. She told me to use my imagination. I am pretty sure that I told her some very odd things, because I certainly had an imagination.

I started going to counseling, but it just did not help. I felt like they never knew what they were talking about, and I hated having to talk to a white person. I felt as though they had this picture-perfect life and that there was no way they could relate to me or what I was experiencing. How could someone help me if they had never experienced the things that I had experienced? As I grew older, the pain grew deeper, and so did my anger. Sometimes I was so depressed that I felt like I was going to have a panic attack, and my heart would stop beating.

One day I got a plastic bag, put it over my head, and tried to suffocate myself, but as much as I felt like dying, that was not the way that I wanted to go. So on my last gasp for breath, I took the bag off of my head and decided to cause a fuss with my foster mom. It was not long before she gave her thirty days' notice, and I was placed in another home. I was only in this home for one day before I ran.

This time, I ran to my aunt's house and begged her to let me stay. She was also a drug addict and loony as a duck. Her trailer was infested with roaches, and at night, you had to sleep with your ears plugged to keep the roaches from crawling into them. She agreed to let me stay, but told me that I better not bring any heat to her house. I promised that I would be on my best behavior and make sure that I was not seen. I needed some clothes and other things, so I had no choice but to call Carlos. He was there at the drop of a dime. He always took care of me and made sure that my needs were met. He was disappointed that I did not call him sooner, but he promised me that he would never hit me again. He got everything that I needed and also got me pregnant. One day I was hanging in my old neighborhood, and I ran into my granddad. He immediately called the police on me, and I took off running. I climbed in a ditch through one of those gray tunnels and stayed there for hours. I cried and thought, "This is no type of life for me." It was freezing cold, and I felt all alone. When I finally knew the coast was clear I hitched a ride back to my aunt's, and the police were there, waiting for me. I tried to run, but it was too late. Officer Peterson caught me and took no time placing me in handcuffs. He asked me several questions about my boyfriend, Carlos, and I looked at him as though he was crazy. I told him I would never tell him anything. He told me if I was running drugs with him, I would go away for a long time. But I did not care what he said. I was placed in detention again, but this time it was not for long. My social worker agreed to allow me to stay with my aunt, especially since I was pregnant. So, a week later, I was released to her but still in the custody of social services. They told me this would be a trial basis. That trial did not last long. Carlos appeared to be happy about the baby, but I was not. I knew nothing about being a parent or raising a child. He was never there unless he wanted some ass, and his excuse was always that he was out making money so that he could buy the baby things. I lost the baby about two months into my pregnancy.

I cried, but it was the best thing that could have happened to me, because I knew nothing about being a parent and knew that I did not have patience. Carlos was pissed and thought that I did it on purpose. But I did not care what he thought, because he was always in the streets. The only time I saw him was when he wanted some pussy or a punching bag. After I lost the baby, my cousin and I hit the streets hard, and that pissed off my aunt. She was always saying that I was a bad influence on her daughter. That would piss me off, because her daughter was sneaky and screwing far more boys than I was. My aunt was cool sometimes, but when she was drunk and high, she would go off the deep end and want to put me out and would call my social worker and probation officer.

The only time we could keep her quiet was when Carlos would give her a hit of some crack or some money. One day, my cousin and I got into a really big argument that led to a fight. My cousin made a big scene and told her mom that I tried to kill her. My aunt told me that I had to get out of her house, and I was no longer wanted there. She had already contacted my social worker, and she was on her way to pick me up to transport me to another home. When she arrived, I was pissed off and highly upset. I begged my aunt not to make me leave, but she proclaimed that she could not handle me and that I had to grow up, find my own identity, and get some help. She made it very clear that she could not have me in her house, fighting her daughter. My social worker just stood there, and I cussed her out. She had no remorse and acted as though she did not care about how I felt. She had brought another social worker assistant out with her whom I had a great deal of respect for. Mr. Greg was the best. He always knew what to say to me so that I would calm down. I never disrespected him, and I could always keep it real. He talked to me and told me I needed to calm down or my worker was going to call the police. He reminded me that I did not want to go back to detention. My social worker, on the other hand, reminded me that if she needed to, she would call the police. I hated her with a passion, and I always vowed that I would never be a social worker and take people's kids. I begin packing my little rags and crying, secretly wishing that I had a mother who was lost and who would eventually come and find me and rescue me from all the mean people who were treating me badly. As we were leaving, my aunt wished me luck, but my cousin never uttered one word to me. As we were walking to the car, everything in my bones said run and I think Mr. Greg saw it all over my face. He told me, "Angel, it's not worth it." I got in the car and wept the entire time.

As we drove, I noticed that we were not going far, and we turned into a familiar neighborhood. I asked where we were going, and they told me that I was going to stay with the Clemons. A part of me was relieved that I knew them, but I also thought, *"How in the hell are they going to raise me if they already have a daughter who was off the chain"*.

Well, we got to the house, and, of course, I refused to get out of the car. I sat there, crying as though I had lost my best friend. I had moved so much all my life, I never knew what to expect from these foster parents. Every foster parent was different, and each one greeted me differently. I remember Greg talking to me and Mr. Clemons coming to the car and telling me to come inside and not to act as though I did not know him. I smiled and got out of the car. I told them that my things needed to sit outside, because I did not want the roaches to be in their house. I sat on the sofa, still weeping, and I gave Ms. Clemons a hug. After all, she was the mom of my best friend, who I use to run with real hard in the streets. Hell, it was her daughter who taught me how to smoke weed and gave me my first joint. However, even though I knew them, I still did not feel comfortable being in their house. I had not seen them in a long time, and in the past, every time I saw them; I would be at their house, high and passed out in a room or trying to eat up everything. We talked about the rules and what there expectations were, and eventually, my social worker and Greg left. It was amazing, because *as much as we hate our social workers, and we want to blame them for our messed-up lives, when they place us and leave, a part of us feels as though they are leaving us too.* So as they drove off, I cried some more. Even though this placement disrupted on the account of me it was one of my best placements. I never was hungry, and Pastor Eddie laid my foundation and assisted in shaping the person I am today. Mr. Clemons was a pastor, and the one rule that he stood by was going to church; it was not an option. I thank him for that, because it gave me a revelation. He was one man I never heard raise his voice or show any favoritism. It was just that I was too far gone into the streets to be redeemed in such a short time. The most difficult part about this placement was trying to respect Ms. Clemons, because this was my friend's mother, and we did not always get along. This was primarily because I wanted to do what I wanted to do, and I wanted to have my way. It was not long before Carlos was back in the picture, and he was not allowed at the house at all. So I was always sneaking out with him or just breaking curfew. During this stay in foster care, I also became really close with the principal from my school. There was something about her I always had respect for. She was the only one who could get me back on task. Instead of suspending me, she would make me sit in her office whenever I got in trouble. While I was with the Clemons, we had disagreements, because I did not want anyone telling me what to do and I hated going to church. I was angry with God, because I felt no child should ever have to experience what I had at such a young age. I don't remember exactly what happened the one day I demanded to leave this placement. It was not the first time, but this time I was very serious and ready to go. I was willing to be moved to a different placement. I knew that if my social worker did not move me then, I was going to run.

I called my social worker and demanded she find me another placement. She would not listen to anything that I had to say, and I remember cursing her out and threatening to whip her ass and slamming down the phone in her ear. A few days later, I was served with a warrant for curse and abuse and making threats over the phone. I packed my stuff, called Carlos, and bounced. I knew that I would get locked up if I had any other charges. I thought, *that bitch must really hate me to take charges out on me because I cursed at her over the phone.* I learned something new every day, because I did not know that it was a criminal offense to curse at someone over the phone.

Being with Carlos was the worst. I never knew where we were going to stay. We were always getting kicked out of hotels or sleeping over at some crack head's house, but I always felt safe that he would not let anyone but himself harm me. I stayed on the run for a long time, living place to place and always having to hide from the police. I kept in touch with Ms. Rigell, who was my school principal. She always tried to convince me to turn myself in, but I would not do it. I was afraid of what might happen. I thought for sure that this time they would send me far away. One day, I found myself in a hotel and really high. I was with some of my girls, and these guys were trying to take advantage of me. I sprayed everyone with mace, got the car keys, and me and my girls left the hotel room full speed! I had no real idea of how to drive, but I was going to learn that day. It was a crack head's car. We jumped in and took off. We drove down the road, laughing and having a good time. I was speeding, and as I came around the corner, I tried to hit the brakes, but the car would not stop. We hit a ditch and flipped three times. We didn't receive one broken bone or even a scratch. We tried to run, but we did not get far, because we were identified by several of the people who lived in the neighborhood. My two friends went home, and I caught several other charges and was sent back to detention. After I did well there, I was stepped down to less secure. I was stupid and making very poor choices.

I allowed this boy in less secure to talk me into running. I was placed in Petersburg, knew nothing about the city, but ran anyway. We were chased by dogs. I ran into all types of bushes, and I have to admit I was scared. After escaping those big-ass dogs on those train tracks, I did not want to run anymore. I told Scoot that he was going to have to go without me. He begged me to stay, but I was hungry, bruised, scared, and had no idea where we were. I told him good-bye and wished him luck. I never saw him again. I flagged down the first police officer, and I was transported right back to Crater detention home. I was shook up for a while, because those dogs scared the mess out of me. It was about four Dobermans that had chased us, and it was nothing but God who had saved us, but I never knew I could run so fast! I was sentenced to about thirty more days in detention and then I went to court. To my luck, I was released and told not to step foot back in the courtroom or I was going back upstate indefinitely. Judge Hoover made it clear that he did not want to see me anymore. To my surprise, my social worker did not transport me to my new placement. Instead, my probation officer did. I kept asking where was I going, but she would not tell me. We had a long talk, and she told me that I had a lot of potential and that I was letting it go to waste. She asked me to please make better decisions and that the judge really saw something in me. She admitted that she thought that I should have been sent back upstate, but she wanted to give me another chance because of the cards that life had already dealt me. She knew that I was angry, but she said she still saw the little girl inside me. She then began to tell me that she would be leaving soon to fulfill her dream of becoming an attorney. She was moving to another state. I cried profusely; I knew that I would never get another probation officer like her.

We pulled up to a very nice neighborhood and an even nicer house. Standing in the doorway was my principal, with tears in her eyes. I looked at my probation officer, and she, too, had tears in her eyes. I said, "She is not a foster parent." She said, "She is now. She came to social services and asked what she had to do to have you stay with her." I got out of the car and hugged her. We all sat down and talked. It was an amazing house, and it felt so comfortable—so comfortable that I was nervous. I had never felt this way before. My probation officer explained to her that my new probation officer would most likely be Ms. Hills. This did not make me happy, because she was a mean woman. I had seen her in court on several occasions, and she was known for sending people upstate. I was placed on house arrest again, but this time without the bracelet. I was pissed about this, because I was an addict and needed a joint. Before my probation officer left, I asked Ms. Rigell if she knew my history. They both said yes, and I asked her if she still wanted me.

She still said yes! This made me very happy, but I was sad that Ms. Mills was leaving. She promised to keep in contact. I cried and said my final good-byes. Then Mrs. Rigell introduced me to her son; I already knew her husband, because he was a substitute at the school. She showed me to my room, which was immaculate. I fell onto the big bed, and I wished that this was my real family. At school, things were kind of weird because I was living with my principal, but none of the other kids knew, except my close friends.

I was still testing the waters because it was just in me. A person does not change overnight. My punishment would spill over to the house, and this would piss me off. I could never watch anything I wanted to on TV, because it was not allowed; this also pissed me off. She would even monitor whom I was talking to on the phone, and I had a phone curfew. I was not use to these rules. I had not seen or heard from Carlos in long time, and I thought about him occasionally. So I tried to find him. She was always taking me on trips to meet her family. She never put me in respite; I was treated like family. But sometimes she made me sick, because she would always correct the way that I talked and say, "We don't use slang in this family," or, "We don't eat that way in this family." It was something about her that I loved but hated at the same time. It was the love and the hugs and the dinners together that made me feel funny. This feeling made me uncomfortable, and I just did not like it at all. One day I asked if I could walk to the store because I seen some friends on our way home. She told me no because I was on house arrest. So I asked if I could invite them over, and, of course, she said no to that as well and quickly told me it was not up for discussion. This added fuel to my fire. We got into an argument, and as soon as she turned her back, I jolted for the door. I was tired of living this way, and I needed some weed. I wanted to hang and chill and see what was going on in the hood. Well, before I made in down the lane, she was in her truck and following me. She got out of the truck and told me to get in. She told me that I was no longer going to run every time I got mad. I told her to leave me alone, and she told me that I had five seconds to get in the truck. I told her that she was not going to do anything, because she could not touch me. She began counting, and I began walking. The next thing I knew, she had grabbed me by my shirt and was yanking me to the truck. I told her to get off me, and as I began to break loose, she threw me onto the backseat. I began to kick, scream, and cry. I screamed, "Why do you care? Just leave me alone." She was pinning me down and crying, saying, "I love you, and you have been through enough. I am not going to let you do this to yourself." I told her I wanted to die, and I struggled some more. But she never let me up. She cried with me and told me that she loved me and that she was going to love me through all my pain. I would one day find out that she would keep her promise. Eventually, I stopped struggling. She got off me, and we went back to the house as though nothing happened. She told me to clean up and prepare for breakfast. At the time, my grandma Daisy was at the house, and she came in and asked me why was I giving my mom Gwen such a hard time? She told me that, one day, my name was going to be in the spotlight, and it was not going to be for a crime.

This family really did show me love, but the streets kept calling. That night I ran away. I ran back to what made me comfortable: the hood and the drugs! I called Mom Gwen this time and told her that I was sorry for hurting her, but it was too late to give me a family. I told her the streets were my home. My grandma Daisy picked up the phone and said, "Baby, we praying for you."

This time, I was running hard and doing whatever I had to do to survive. I began dancing and letting men do disgusting things to me just to get some money so that I could eat. I was sleeping in cars and sometimes under trees. I missed my warm house, and I wanted to go back, but I knew that I was already violated and was going to be sent upstate. So I decided to take full advantage of being out in the streets. I had even started this little gang called the Baby Bottles. It was stupid, because when it came down to it, everyone was for him- or herself. I was hurting a lot of people, but mainly myself. I kept in contact with Mom Gwen, and she told me that she was going to be moving to Florida. She had been offered a position that she could not turn down. This pissed me off, because she said that she would always be there for me. I thought *how you can be there for me in Florida? I felt abandoned again.*

At this point, I was at rock bottom. I remember being in a crack house, and this old guy offered me some crack. I was so out of it, so alone, and so tired. I just wanted life to end. I had vowed that I would never use any other drug other than weed because of what it had done to my whole family, but this night I just no longer cared. I was sitting on the bed, and he gave me the pipe. I put it to my mouth and lit the lighter. Then I heard something screaming my name. I threw it on the bed and took off running, I ran so fast I had no idea where I was running to, but I was running for dear life. I never knew who called my name, but I thank God for divine intervention. I was already addicted to marijuana and I did not need any additional addictions.

I stayed on the streets a few more days. I was running with Carlos when I could, but he was also on the run, so we did not see each other often. It was getting colder, and my aunt would sometimes let me sleep in her truck, but it was still cold. I was tired of this living, and I needed a safe haven. So I got really high one day and went to my probation officer's office. From there, I went straight to detention. I could not believe that I was going back to Christiansburg detention center. When I got there, some of the staff told me that they knew that I would be back one day, and they reminded me of how I cursed them out when I left. There was no need to apologize, because I had to go straight to lockdown. I was pissed. After all this time, I still had to do my time for something I had done over a year ago. Anyway, I did ten days' lockdown and was allowed to come out of my cell. This time, I was on my best behavior. I was always looking to try and find an escape route, but there was none.

Eventually, my court date came, and to my surprise, the judge overturned the recommendation that I be sent upstate. My social worker at the time was pissed. She stated that the agency was unable to identify a home that was willing to take me because of my behavior. The Judge told her it was her job to find someone. So I had to stay at the agency for hours while they worked on a placement, and my social worker was furious! Eventually, I was told that I would be going to a group home in Richmond, and I thought anything was better than being in detention. The drive was a long one, and when I got there, it looked like a huge campus that housed hundreds of kids. I was checked in, and all the rules were given to me. I met my roommate and was left without a plan. I knew that I had to go back to court in a month, so I vowed to be on my best behavior. For the most part, I did well while I was placed in this group home—with the exception of getting caught smoking cigarettes. Also, I did not do well in school. I hated school, because I felt as though I was just not competent; I had never really gone to school consistently. I was embarrassed about being in school, and I would get pissed if the teacher called on me and asked me a question. I wanted to talk to my social worker about exploring the possibility of going to live with another aunt, but she never returned my phone calls. So, when it was time for me to go to court, I vowed to make the drive miserable for her.

When my court date came, my social worker was running late. I was in class, and no one would give me any answers, so I got very angry and walked out of the school building and began heading to the cottage.

They would not unlock the door, so I took my foot and attempted to kick it in. As I was kicking the door, I broke the glass. They responded by putting me in restraints and placing me in the timeout room.

Shortly afterward, my social worker arrived. I called her several names. She kept a smirk on her face, as though she knew I was going to get locked up. We had a very long drive before we reached the courthouse, and we did not say one word to each other. I always wondered why she disliked me. I knew that I was disrespectful child, but I expected her to know that I was a child in pain. As we entered the court, she walked ahead of me. She could not wait to report to the judge what I had done and that she suspected that the group home was going to file charges for destruction of property. The judge asked me why I did it, and I explained to him that I was nervous and anxious about court because no one had told me anything. Again, I was given yet another chance, and I knew that this pissed off my social worker and probation officer. I walked out of the courtroom proud. I did not want to go back to that group home, but it was better than being locked up; at least I had a little freedom. Well, when it, was time to leave I was full of smirks and destined to piss off my social worker. We got into the van, and I smiled and said, "You thought you were going to get rid of me, didn't you?" She never responded, so I turned on the radio. She turned it off. I turned it on, and she turned it off. As I went to turn the radio back on, she smacked my hand. I raised my fist to hit her, and she quickly turned around and headed back to the courtroom, stating that I had assaulted her. I said, "I did not assault you, but I will show you assault." As we pulled up to the courtroom she jumped out of the van as though she was so afraid of me. I knew what her motive was, but I did not care. I got out of the van and started walking. I thought about running, but the truth was I had nowhere to go, and I was tired of being on the streets and not knowing what was going to happen to me or where I was going to lay my head.

While I was walking, a sheriff came up to me and told me that I needed to head back to the court. I told him to mind his own business; I was not doing anything to anyone, and I was not going anywhere. He told me again that I needed to turn around, and I told him to go to hell. Before I knew it, he grabbed my shoulder, and I started swinging. I think that day I let go of every piece of anger I had in me! I went off in front of that courtroom, and before I knew it, several officers were on me. I was fighting them all until I could not fight anymore. They had me in the air, carrying me through the courtroom. I was spitting and cursing the entire way. They threw me in a holding cell, like I was not a child. As soon as they threw me, I spit at them and continued to curse them. One sheriff told me to calm down, and then Sheriff Cookie came and talked to me. I respected her, so I listened, but I was fuming. I knew that I was surely to go upstate after assaulting a police officer. So I figured what the hell. I was going out with a bang. I knew that I was going to have to be arraigned, so when it was time for them to come and place me in shackles, I stood in the corner like a bull with its nostrils flaring and I charged them with everything I had left in my body. I guess you can say they earned that paycheck that day! (***It's not funny, but it is funny to reflect back on how angry and crazy I once was***) This time they handcuffed me and shackled my feet. I went back in front of Judge Hoover with rage in my eyes, and he simply said, "Committed upstate indefinitely." I cursed my social worker to the end, and she had a smirk on her face the entire time. I was angry with myself, because I let her win. I was so angry that I could not cry anymore.

Back Upstate

This time, I was placed in a detention center in Loudon County until I was to be transported to RDC (Upstate). During my stay in Loudon County, I got into a lot of trouble, but I met some great counselors. When I first met, counselor Rob, and counselor Sherry, we did not hit it off well. They stayed on my ass for everything, and I was always getting locked down for something. I remember getting into a fight and being placed in some restraints. Every time I moved, they tightened up on my feet and arms. I thought this was abuse and that no child should have to go through this. I was placed in a small room with a camera that watched everything that I did. They justified this by saying that I was under suicide watch. It pissed me off and violated me; I had no privacy, not even to use the restroom, but I got a kick out of letting them see me wipe my ass. I stayed in this detention for a while before I was transported upstate. I hated visitation time. No one ever came to visit me, and I never had anyone to call. When I left this place, I was so sad, and I cried for days. It had become home to me, and I was use to the staff and had grown pretty close to some of the residents. Counselor Sherry promised me that she would keep in touch, and she kept her promise.

When I got back upstate, not much had changed. Some of the same residents were there as the last time that I had left. We still wore the same orange jumpsuits and had to be shackled to each other every time we left the cottage. I had no idea where my future was going, and I had begun to give up on life. So I decided to make this place home and adjust to the best of my ability. One day I was feeling down and out, and I got a letter from counselor Sherry. She sent me a poem by Maya Angelou. She told me that despite what cards life had dealt me, I was a phenomenal woman. Sherry had kept her promises. She said she would always be there for me, and actions always speak louder than words. I felt as though I was hitting rock bottom, and this letter really picked me up and encouraged me. The next week I got a letter from Mom Gwen. I was shocked and amazed. I had not heard from her in a while. She was in Florida and doing well. I cried the entire time that I read the letter. I received a letter from her almost every week; they were really encouraging. In her eyes I was still her daughter and she reminded me that I had a family that was praying for me.

While upstate, I tried so hard to stay out of trouble, but it was difficult. When you are locked up, you are locked up with people from all walks of life. You really learn about different cultures, and the way some of these girls were, you had to be ready to fight at any time. There was no sense in backing down, because if you did, you would surely become someone's bitch! I was in a room with four other girls, and for the most part, we were all cool. But two of them were gay, so we always had some type of conflict. One day, I called my social worker and asked her if it was possible to go back to my dad and she told me no and did not give an explanation other than that placement was no longer an option. I had been upstate for several months and had no idea of what was going to happen to me and then I got a visit from someone who was supposed to be my new social worker. She asked me if I was interested in moving to Florida and I immediately said no. She then told me that there were no other alternatives and that Mrs. Rigell had requested that I live in Florida with her. I was vexed, because she did all this behind my back.

My social worker went on to explain that I could be upstate for a very long time, but it would be possible that I could get my sentenced shortened if I agreed to go to another state. She went on to say that it would be almost impossible to find a placement for me due to my extensive history and my age. I asked her if I could think about it, and she told me that I did not have much time because they needed to begin the paperwork. She said that she would call me in a few weeks. I wrote Mrs. Rigell and asked her why she didn't tell me her plans. She responded by saying that she was being led by God, and it was time that I had a home and a family. She was always talking to me about the importance of permanency. She told me that they wanted to be the one to give it to me. She told me how much she loved me, and she was missing one thing: her daughter. I asked her, "Do you know that I have problems and that I am crazy?" She told me the enemy was making me believe that I was crazy and then she laughed and told me that she was crazy to. I told her that I had several tests run, and they said that I had borderline personality disorder, but she did not seem to care. I did not think I was worthy of being loved and I did not understand how anyone could love a bitter, disrespectful child like me.

When my social worker called, I told her that I was willing to go. Within the next two months, I had a release date. I was picked up by two workers and transported to Richmond airport. I had no clothes except for what was on my back, and my hair was a mess. I was afraid to fly, but it felt good to be free. When I left upstate this time, some of the workers said, "We'll see you again real soon." Others wished me luck and told me I was afforded a wonderful opportunity and to take full advantage of it. There were some negative, nasty counselors who worked upstate; some of the counselors in detention would intentionally try to provoke you so they could restrain you. I never understood their motives other than it being an adrenaline rush. I promised God that if he got me out this time, I was never going to return.

A New Atmosphere in a different state

I will never forget the day that I boarded that plane. I cried because I felt as though I was leaving something behind. I cried because I thought life was not fair and that this should not be happening to me and what did I do to deserve this treatment? I cried because I was afraid of new beginnings and had no idea what I would be walking into. I cried because I was going to miss my girls' upstate, the ones I felt as though I left behind. My flight to Florida was fairly quiet. I thought about my dad, my sister, and even a little thought of the woman who was supposed to be my mom. I wondered what they were doing and if anyone thought about me or even knew that I was going to Florida. So many thoughts ran through my mind, and I remember sinking in my seat and the tears flowing. When the flight landed, butterflies were in my stomach. I had not seen Mom Gwen in a long time. I did not know what to expect, and I must admit that I looked like a little bum and felt ashamed. I did not feel pretty, and I did not want her to see me looking so bad, because I thought she wouldn't love me anymore. I had on some jogging pants and a T-shirt, and my hair had not been done in months because as I stated earlier there was no such thing as a perm or a hairdresser upstate. When I walked off that plane, I met

Mom Gwen, crying and hugging me tightly, and another small, petite, white lady who was also crying. I learned that she was my new social worker, so I wondered why in the hell she was crying. I continued to stare at them and wonder what all the tears were about. We took several pictures, which I was not comfortable about. I was not use to taking pictures at all. They asked me where my other things were, and I held my head down and said, "I don't have anything else. It's just me." I saw the look on their face that said "How dare they send her down here with absolutely nothing except the clothes on her back," but my mom Gwen played it off and said, "That's okay. The most important thing is that my baby is home, and all that other stuff we will take care of later."

So we left the airport and headed to what was supposed to become my new home. On entering the house, my brother Stevie greeted me, along with his dad, Mr. Rigell. I had not seen Stevie in years, and he had grown a lot. Mr. Rigell still looked the same, and he gave me a big hug and told me he was making my favorite meal, fried chicken and mac and cheese. That made me smile because upstate fried chicken was unheard of. There were balloons hanging and welcome home signs everywhere. I wondered what was wrong with this woman and why did she love me more than my own mother! It was a weird feeling, but I always felt safe when I was in her presence. It was a piece of me that wished she was my biological mother. I would secretly wonder how my life would be if she would have had me from birth.

We sat down and discussed rules. Ms. Mienke (my new social worker) was talking with Mom Gwen about paperwork and then she began to tell me what my expectations were. She told me that I would have to complete anger management and that I would meet my probation officer at some point tomorrow. I was expected to attend school and refrain from all uses of drugs. I thought *whatever*. The first question that came out of my mouth was when I would be allowed to go home to Virginia. Ms. Mienke quickly reminded me that I would have to complete all the rules of my probation successfully and get adjusted to my new home before we could talk about visiting Virginia. The first night was very difficult for me, and even though I knew in my heart that I was safe, it was still not home. This house was big, clean, and peaceful. There were no drunks lurking around, no fighting, no cursing, just a fresh aroma and a feeling of peace. As my mom Gwen took me to my room, my bed was soft, clean, and cozy. It was nice to take a real shower and be able to put on some real pajamas. My mom Gwen felt the need to tuck me in, and even though I tried to act as though I did not like it, the truth was I loved every moment. She cried as she tucked me in and told me how happy she was that I was home. She told me that now everything was complete. She always made sure that she reassured me that I was safe from harm and that no one was going to hurt me anymore. I did not cry while she was in the room, but I felt very special, and I believed her when she said I was safe. After she left the room, I cried myself to sleep, because I did not know what the next day or weeks would look like. I kept waiting for this lady to stop loving me or to ship me back to Virginia or to say something nasty to me. But it never happened. ***This lady, whom I came to love and trust, spoke life unto me through prayer and commitment and broke all the bondages that had me bound.***

The next couple of weeks we spent in the stores buying me clothes and shoes and getting me all the things that a child should have. I would always try and have an outburst about something, but it was very difficult, because Mom Gwen could calm any storm with very few words. I would get angry because I was use to dressing like a tomboy and wearing my pants big and sagging, but that was not allowed in her house. She would make me so angry, because I also liked to wear white tees, but she would always tell me that young girls don't dress like young

Angel Bartlett

boys. No matter what I said, she always meant what she said and would never argue with a child. When it was time for me to begin school, there were many problems. I did not get along with the other students, and compared to my classmates, I was behind in so many areas. I would create problems so that I could be dismissed from class and sent to the office. I was embarrassed, because learning was difficult for me, and I was always too ashamed to ask for any help. This made my mother very upset, because she was the principal at the neighboring school and was well known in the community. But she was never ashamed of "her baby"—that is what she called me. She would punish me by taking the phone, which was my only connection to my friends back in Virginia.

Eventually, I made some friends in Florida, and they were not the right friends. My mom had a spirit of discernment, and if she discerned anything about you, you were not allowed over to our house. This was very nerve-racking, because she discerned something about most of my friends. The funny part is, she was always right. If I had listened to her, I would have saved myself a lot of problems and heartache. There continued to be struggles with me in school, and eventually I got into a fight and was suspended, but because I had been doing everything else that I was suppose to do, I did not receive a violation of parole. My mom Gwen made me work at her school during my suspension, and that was miserable, but there was no such thing as lying in the bed and sleeping all day. Florida was difficult for me, because I did not have the liberty to do what I wanted when I wanted. Structure was difficult for me to adjust to. I tried very hard not to disrespect my mom Gwen, but it was difficult, because I was naturally a rude and wounded child. But no matter what I did or said, she never threatened to kick me out, and she never treated me any differently. She would punish me and then we would move on to the next thing. I remember one day Stevie asked me why I called Mom Ms. Rigell. My mom Gwen always knew when

I did not know what to say, and she always had the ability to say the right things and make me feel comfortable. At this point in my life, I did not even refer to my biological mother as Mom; I called her by her first name. Even though Ms. Rigell was the closest thing to a mom that I ever had, the word sent chills up my spine. But eventually, after all the hell I put her through, it came naturally. I don't remember the day that I called her mom, but I know that once I began, I never stopped. One day I was in the kitchen, and I was really depressed and missing Virginia, and I felt as though I wanted to die. I often had days that I would become depressed, and my mom always knew. She tried to keep me active, but sometimes a spirit of depression would just overwhelm me.

On this particular day, I had been seeking attention by being rude, but it was not working. So I began rambling through the kitchen, looking for pills. As I found them, I popped them quickly into my mouth. My mom got off of the sofa, came into the kitchen, and restrained me on the floor, taking her hands and prying the pills out of my mouth. She began praying over me, and we lay on that kitchen floor for hours, both of us crying. She kept telling me, "Let it out, let it out." How could a child have so much pain and anger to the point where she just wants to end her life? I had that much pain, and sometimes I was so sad that I thought life would be better if I was dead. I loved my mom Gwen, but I was use to so much chaos that having a normal life did not feel right and made me even more depressed. I think it was because when drama occurred or I was drugged up, I did not have to face the facts that I was abused, abandoned, neglected, and not loved by my parents. I was able to escape with the drugs and with the drama. But while I was in Florida, I had to come to grips with the fact that I was a wounded child who needed to be healed, or I was going to kill myself or someone was going to kill me.

After my suicide attempt was over, our day proceeded as normal. She never called anyone; we dealt with everything in house, and she always told me that was how a family was supposed to operate. I would often say to her, "Go ahead and call the people now and tell them that I have to leave," but she would respond with a simple, "Angel, my child, you are home, and no one is going to take you anywhere." Sometimes I would get so angry with her that I would just yell at her, hoping that she would change her mind and turn her back on me, but no matter how difficult I was, she stuck by me through everything. There were so many times when I would be in my room at night and thinking of killing myself, because regardless of how much I felt loved by this woman, I always had a void that could not be filled. I had to understand something that I was too young to comprehend, and whenever I tried to figure it out, a pain would enter my stomach that made me feel so bad that I just wanted to die. My mom Gwen would come in my room at night, lie beside me, and cry with me, always letting me know that I would get through this and that I was more than a conquer! Sometimes she would come into my room and we would just cry and not speak one word to each other. Somehow, she always knew what I needed the most. Sometimes I would cry myself to sleep, and when I would wake, she would be by my side, praying over me. I knew there were times that I hurt my mom deeply by the mean things that I said, but she loved me anyway and always stayed committed to me.

Once I got involved with a man who was twenty-five years my senior. This sent her over the deep edge. I was skipping school to be with him, and I thought that I was in love. Somehow, my mom found out, and she contacted him personally and told him that if he did not stay away from me, she would make sure the jail was sat on top of him. I finally got in touch with him one day at school, and he told me what she had said. He told me that he was not going to see me anymore, and this sent me off the deep end. I was so angry that if I could have caught on fire from being so angry, I would have burned to death. I tried to call my mom several times. I never got an answer, but I left her several nasty messages. When I got home, I tore up my momma's house; I snatched out the phones, and turned over sofas. She never budged. She sat very calmly and told me that I was searching for love in all the wrong places, and what did a forty-year-old man want with an immature teenager? I told that she did not understand and that I was going to continue to see him. I hated her for this, but in the long run, I thanked her because he was a big-time drug dealer. He eventually went to jail, and if she had not intervened, I probably would have been right there with him, because I always considered myself a ride-or-die chick. It took a long time for me to get over this man and an even longer time for me to forgive and understand my mom Gwen, but eventually we were able to move on, because there was always some new drama brewing with me. I was doing everything that I was supposed to do, with the exception of getting into trouble at school. For me, that was very good and was an excellent milestone.

I never stopped asking about going back to Virginia, and the day finally came when I was allowed to have a visit in Virginia. I had been begging my workers back in Virginia to let me come home for at least for a visit, but they always had excuses about supervision and who would keep me. I was finally able to get my aunt to agree to a visit with her. She was the only aunt I had who was not addicted to drugs. So I was given two weeks to visit in Virginia. My mom Gwen cried profusely, but I promised her I was going to make good choices. At the airport, you would have thought mom Gwen would never see me again, but when I looked in her eyes, my heart told me that I would come back. I reminded her that I was still on parole and that I was not going back upstate for anyone or anything. She smiled a little and told me she would see me soon. I hugged her and my brother and went on my way. Getting on the plane and flying back to Virginia, I had several emotions, ranging from butterflies to excitement. And I wanted to see everyone, including Carlos. Well, when I got to the airport, I met my new social worker, and my old social worker accompanied her. She did not look thrilled to see me, but she managed to muster up a fake smile, and I mustered a fake smile in return. My new social worker looked frightened, and I told her that I was not as bad as they probably told her I was. She looked at me as though she could not believe I read her mind! We left the airport, and needless to say, the old worker started in on reminding me of what I was not supposed to do and when I was supposed to return to Florida. I immediately told her to chill out and that I was not going to run away and give her the satisfaction of sending me back upstate. I was very happy to see my aunt, but, of course, she had to begin with all her rules. She also let me know that she would not hesitate to call the police on me. I thought, *damn, for all this I could have stayed in Florida*. I felt as though no one wanted me to be in Virginia, including my aunt. My aunt assured the workers that she would have me back at the agency on time so that I could be transported to the airport. She also assured them that she would call them if she had any problems. I knew she was telling the truth. When they left, I was like, "Dang, Aunt Peggy, you act like you don't want me here," but she said, "No, I just want you to stay out of trouble." I told her she did not have to act like that in front of those white folks.

Well, I could not wait to get on the phone and call everyone I knew and make plans. My aunt did not mind me going out, but she was adamant that I have no contact with Carlos. Of course, Carlos had already heard through the grapevine that I was going to be in town, so it was not long before he came to the hood looking for me. I was happy to see him, and we showed each other love, but I told him I was not allowed to be with him, but he was not trying to hear it. I missed him, but I was not about to ruin my stay for him, and I was no longer willing to have him whip my ass. Those days where officially over, and I told him that. He was pissed off and promised me that he would not hurt me or put his hands on me. He begged me to spend time with him, but I told him no. He got angry and grabbed me by my arms, but immediately apologized. I told him if I was caught with him, my aunt would report it to my social worker. This vexed Carlos, but he did not want me to get into any trouble, so he stopped putting so much pressure on me. One night I was at my aunt's and the phone ring. It was Carlos, and he said that he had to have some of my time and this shit was dumb and why was I allowing people to keep us apart. He told me that he was outside and to come and talk to him. As I proceeded to go outside, my aunt said, "If you go outside, I am calling the police." I tried to explain to her that I was only going to talk to him, but she did not want to hear it. So I packed my stuff like a dummy and told her that I did not want to stay with her anymore and that I made a mistake coming to visit her. She immediately got on the phone and called the police, but I was in the wind. I told Carlos, "Let's bounce." I called my social worker the next day and told her that I was okay, but I could not stay with my aunt anymore. They told me that they had moved my plane ticket, and I had forty-eight hours to be at the airport or I would be violated. I hung up the phone, pissed and mad as hell. I wanted to say fuck it, but I knew that I could not do that, because I was tired of living a life on the run and had came so far I did not want to regress. Carlos promised to take care of me and begged me not to go, but I explained to him that I no longer wanted to live a life on the run and that I was going to complete parole and move back to Virginia. He cried and begged me to stay, but I could not. I told him if he loved me, he would encourage me to do right and wait for me until I could come back to Virginia. I called my mom in Florida later that night, and she told me that she had been praying for me. I told her that I tried to do right, but my aunt was tripping from the time I landed in Virginia. She reminded me of how much I had accomplished and begged me not to throw it all away. I told her that I was going to be at the airport on time. When it was time to go, Carlos gave me some money, and I caught the cab to the airport. It was the hardest thing to do but the best decision I could have made. Both social workers were there, and the only thing I said was, "I want to come back home to Virginia, so please start working on finding me a placement or preparing me to be emancipated." I had mixed emotions about leaving Virginia, but one thing I knew for sure: I never wanted to live a life on the run again!

When I got back to Florida, my mom was livid when she had seen my hair: I had colored it orange. But she was still happy to see me, and I was happy to get back in my bed. The very next day, she bought me some dye and made me color my hair black. I talked with her about wanting to go back to Virginia, and even though she did not think that would be a good idea, she would support me in whatever I wanted to do. She also reminded me that this would always be home. I asked her to move back to Virginia, but she told me there was no way she was leaving this sunny weather to come back to Virginia.

Back to Virginia

It felt good going back to Virginia, knowing that I was no longer on parole and the only person I had to deal with was my social worker. And for the first time in my life, I always knew that I had a place to call home, which was in Florida with my mom Rigell. She cried when I left, and so did I, but she taught me so much while I was there I knew that I would never be the same again. I still had many struggles, but I knew that I wanted more for myself. I had a determination to achieve more than what others thought I would. When I got back to Virginia, I was allowed to go and live with my sister, which was odd. She had her own place and had been doing well, so they set me up there in an independent living situation. I began receiving $644.00 a month as a stipend and was enrolled in the GED program. It was good being with my sister. It was my sister, my cousin, her boyfriend, and her three kids. It was a big change from what I had gotten used to in Florida, but I was determined to make it work. It the meantime, school was a struggle. I hated attending and did not have a lot of help. Carlos had gotten locked up and was given forty-five years in prison, so I did not have him to deal with. I was hurt about his time, but Carlos had done a lot of bad things to and hurt many people. I told Carlos he was not being sentenced for the current charge, but all the pain he had inflicted upon me and so many others

I soon met this guy, and we became very close. I became very close to his mother, and she began to help me with a lot of things. She was a 1st sergeant in the military and big on education. My sister and I were not getting along at all, so I began to spend a lot of time at their house. To my surprise, it was okay when I stayed the night. Sometimes I would call her in the morning, crying because I missed the bus and did not have a ride to class, and she would leave her job and come and take me all the way to school. Her son and I were very close, and I felt like this family was my family, too. My sister was becoming a real bitch, and I hated staying with her and was sick of sleeping on the floor. So, when my boyfriend went off to the military, his family invited me to stay with them for good. They had no problem contacting my social worker and complying with anything in order to be able to receive me in their home. I soon transitioned to their house, and I was so happy. I eventually passed my GED and began working as a waitress at IHOP. While I was living in Florida, I had several different jobs, so obtaining a job was not a difficult task. But I knew working at IHOP or McDonald's was not going to take me where I wanted to go in life. Mom Pettaway, who was now my second mom, was always telling me that I had to go to college or military. I would always get upset and say that no one was going to accept me because I had a GED. That was true to a certain degree, because I got several rejection letters from different Colleges and University's. So finally, Mom Pettaway suggested that I try community college. She basically completed the application for me, and I was accepted. It was the happiest day of my life, but I was still making dumb choices. I was addicted to marijuana and just could not kick the habit. Mom and Poppa Pettaway loved me dearly, but I was beginning to get into more arguments with their son and we had broken up. He was stationed in Georgia and had moved on with his life. They loved me just like their daughter, but it was a difficult relationship, because they were always caught in the middle of our drama. So one day I suggested that I move out and get my own place. I had no independent living skills, but I also did not want to disrespect the people who were helping me so much, and their son was getting on my nerves.

One night they were out of town, and I had their car. I had it out past my curfew, and I almost got killed when someone shot the car with me in it and shot my cousin twice in the arm. They were happy that I was not harmed but naturally pissed about the car. It took several weeks to get the car out of the pound and even longer to get the bullet holes filled. I was afraid to ride in the car, because the people who shot at us were never found. I had nightmares that they were going to come back and kill me, so the car was eventually sold. I never understood why two men would try and kill three females. This incident put a lot of strain on our relationship, but they still supported and loved me. But I was ready to be on my own so against their will, I got an apartment in the projects with a girlfriend. My social worker supported this, and they gave me some assistance from social services. This was the worst decision I could have made, but I had already signed a lease. My house became the party house, and I knew nothing about managing bills.

Through all my dumb mistakes, I had support from two wonderful mothers: Mom Gwen and Mom Pettaway. Mom Pettaway always made sure that I attended school. I will never forget the first day of registration. I was afraid to get out of the car, and she told me to get my black ass out of the car and go and handle my business. I sat in the car for several minutes, crying because I never dreamed that I would be at anyone's college or actually engaging with other students who probably would have never made it in life if they had to walk in my shoes! I was always told that I would be dead or in jail, but thus far, I was proving the critics wrong.

I did not have my apartment long before I moved out and back home with the Pettaways. I could not pay the bills, and I no longer wanted to try. Mom Pettaway welcomed me back home with open arms.

Eventually, my uncle Bill contacted me and told me to submit an application for Saint Paul's College. He told me that he would be able to pull a few strings, because I needed to get out of Newport News. I was a little skeptical, because I had only been in community college for a little while and did not want to get another letter of rejection from another school. But together with Mom Pettaway, I submitted my application and essay, and I was accepted. I would soon be leaving to go to college, a real college I thought.

It was not long before the devil started attacking my mind and making me feel like I was too dumb and smoked too much weed and that I would be the only ghetto person attending college. But none of that mattered. I knew that come January 1, 2000, I had to get out of that house and leave for school or the military. Community college was too close to what was familiar, and it was not working for me. I also no longer wanted to stay with Mom Pettaway, but I had nowhere else to go unless I went back to Florida. Though I missed my mom Gwen, I was not going back to Florida! I knew that I had no worries about paying for anything while I was in college, because social services were going to take care of everything. I had to stay out of trouble and maintain a grade point average of at least 2.5, and everything else would be taken care of. I also was still going to receive my stipend of $644.00. The day before I was supposed to leave for school, I got into an argument with Mom Pettaway, so they did not take me to school, and I did no care. I had come a long way, but I was still a bitter, angry, and sometimes disrespectful child. I was eighteen years old now, but I still carried with me all the anger from my childhood and that is why I was still addicted to marijuana. It made me feel like I was on cloud nine, and I did not care about anything. When I was high I was able to cope with my past and my present! So several of my girlfriends got together and took me to school. The campus was small and full of black people. I was told I was going to be attending a historical black college, but growing up where I did, black people did not go to college so, this was different for me. I was nervous as hell, because I thought these were going to be black people who spoke proper English and came from two-parent homes and had their future planned.

To my surprise, there were several broken people on campus just like me and even more ghetto than I. So I met the dean and was taken to my room. My girls helped me unpack, and to my surprise, they left me with a whole ounce of weed. That made me feel a little better, because when they left, I cried and felt all alone. I walked off campus, rolled me a blunt, and got high as a kite. As I walked back on campus, I met several people who seemed cool. They introduced themselves to me, but I did not want to socialize. I went to my room, and as I walked through the halls, I smelled marijuana. I was very surprised. I thought that I had escaped the ghetto, but it appeared that it had followed me to school. However, I knew that I had to find out who else smoked so that we could be friends. That night I cried myself to sleep and thought, *the ghetto has followed me to school!*

Four Years of College

The next day, I woke up and was still depressed. Depression seemed to follow me everywhere I went. I was starving, so I knew I had to come out of my shell, and I knew I only had one chance to get it right. As each day progressed, I met more people. Some were haters and others became lifelong friends. I struggled with a lot of things, and I always had to spend extra time with my professors because I was behind academically, but the professors were always willing to go beyond the call of duty to help me. I completed my first semester and was even able to go and visit some of my friends on the weekends, because I met a guy who also lived in Newport News. The worst thing I could have done was to continue to smoke weed, but I was addicted, and at the time, I could not kick the habit. Even when I tried, it was hard because everyone that I made friends with smoked.

After completing my first semester, I went home for the summer with my mom Pettaway, and that is what made me realize that God led me to Saint Paul's for a reason: I needed to stay away from the hood that was my past! My first summer home, I was working at a gas station when a woman I didn't know came in. She told me that I had made some threats to her cousin several years back and that she was going to kick my ass! I saw her cousin in the car, and I could not believe that this was coming back to haunt me. This had happened when I was sixteen years old. She asked me what time I got off, and being the person that I am, I told her. I wasn't afraid of anyone. The both of them together were about 500 pounds to my 130 pounds. I called my boy and had him bring me his burner. Then I called my girls and had them meet me at my job. I secretly hoped they did not show up, but to no one's surprise, those bitches were at my job at 5:00 PM on the dot. I had no intentions of shooting her, but I was going to pistol-whip the hell out of her! However, that did not happen, because as I went to pull out the gun, I dropped it and everyone from the hood was outside. My homeboy picked up the gun and stashed it in the woods. So, when she saw that I had a gun but then lost it, this added even more fuel to her fire. She immediately attacked me, and we fought like cats and dogs right outside my job. The only person who caught charges that day was me, and I went to jail. As I sat in that police car, my whole life flashed before me. I saw me losing everything, going to jail, and never being anything in life. I was afraid that I would fail and even more afraid that I was going to disappoint the two women who believed in me when no one else did. The charges were put in the paper, and everything that I had worked so hard for was about to be taken away, because I was too stupid to just walk away and call the police and report the threats that she had made. I asked God to please get me out of this one and to allow me to wake up from this nightmare. I vowed that if I got off this one, I would never look back at my past again, and I would never fight again. By the grace of God, he saved me again, and I beat all charges. As I walked out of the courtroom, I knew that I would never fight again! From that point on, I went to summer school every year and was very mindful of everything that I did. I was determined to beat the odds. ***I needed that incident to occur, because it showed me that I was still angry and that if I***

did not change my ways and forgive people, nothing—including college—was going to save me.

Despite my many challenges in college, I made it. I taught other students how to appreciate their nagging parents and the holidays that they were made to come home because I did not have that. When parents came to school to visit their kids, it was so sad for me, because I did not have that. But I was still determined to make it. College helped me to develop my talents and meet friends who would love me for life and encourage me to pursue my dreams. I turned twenty-one before I graduated, so I aged out of the foster-care system. That was very difficult for me because I was never adopted, and I knew that I could always depend on social services if I had a need. However, after I aged out of care, I had support from wonderful people who continued to support me. My Uncle Bill and Aunt Gail sent me money every month. They paid my rent when I moved off campus for an entire year. They bought me a car and treated me as though I was their biological niece. I felt loved and much supported, even though I did not have my biological mother or father! I had a host of support from my Mom Gwen and her entire family. My social worker always kept in touch with me and helped link me with other resources. I always tell people that if I could still be in care and taking full advantage of those resources, I would. I knew that I was going to be a social worker, and I was going to be better than some of the social workers that I had. I was going to be a voice and advocate for kids in foster care.

On May 11, 2003, I walked across the stage and graduated with my bachelor's in Sociology with a concentration in Criminal Justice. Who would have ever thought? And on my graduation day, I had two mothers, Mom Pettaway and Mom Gwen, with the two happiest smiles. They were my biggest cheerleaders, and I knew that this was only the beginning. I knew that there would still be many challenges, but at this point in my life, I believed in myself and what I was capable of obtaining. I knew that God had equipped me to be strong, and I was ready to face the many challenges that lay ahead waiting for me. My mom Gwen would always tell me that God will never leave you nor forsake you, and I finally understood that concept. Graduating from college was a defining moment, but I was ready for more. I wanted to go all the way. ***I had a attitude like P-Diddy, (can't stop, won't stop)***

Note to Readers

This book is a memoir of my journey through the foster-care system and a very troubled childhood. A memoir is defined as "a record of events based on the writer's personal knowledge". So for the spectator's that will say "well she call her-self saved, but look at all the profanity" I say to you that this is memories of who I use to be! I will not change my life or story for anyone. The GLORY is in the STORY.

Growing up in foster care is very difficult and challenging. I can remember so many days being in the courtroom and not understanding what was going on. Some of the jargon is something that a child will never understand, but he or she should be totally involved with the whole process. In addition, all children need a voice. The saddest part is that even today, most kids in foster care do not know what or who their guardian ad litem—GAL—is. I find it to be very sad when a GAL meets a child the day of court and the only time they speak to the child is when the child is in court. They are supposed to be the child's biggest advocate and know all aspects of what is going on in that child's life. However, they have disappointed me in the past and continue to be disappointing today. As a current social worker I despise working with people like you and when I am interacting with you I pray that

God hold's my tongue and allows me to maintain my professionalism. How can you represent a child and you have never seen where they lay there head? Or you have never had a conversation with them outside of court?

You will notice in this book that a lot of names are not used. That is because they did something that was unethical or contributed to my anger/depression. I eventually lost count of the number of placements that I had in the foster-care system, but what I do know is there are some foster parents who don't need to be foster parents. They only add to the hurt and anger that many of us already have. I have changed a lot of names and identifying details to include certain timelines to protect certain identities. For many events, I relied on documentation from previous social services records. At the end of the book you will find inserts from various court reports, evaluations and etc. The reason for this is to substantiate my life. Some people are in denial about what they did to me and others won't believe that someone could make it through, but documentation does not lie!

I often wonder why some social workers became social workers because I have met some heart-less social workers even in my professional walk. Social workers have no idea what they do to children when they move them because they are angry because the foster parent has challenged them on their work performance. Please note that it is not about you, and sometimes you need to be challenged. Or is it that you need to refer back to your code of ethics? Also, some social workers are quick to move a child because they may have a concern. But how much information do you really have if you only visit once a month, and sometimes you don't even complete your monthly visit. (Oops did I say that?)

To the thousands of children who are in foster care and whose voices are not heard, I promise to be your voice and to say what needs to be said! I urge you to take advantage of the services that are offered to you, mainly the counseling. I wish that I had taken more advantage of the counseling, because as I grew older, I realized that I needed help on my issues of trust and love and I still struggle with forming and maintaining relationships. Even today, I am not perfect, but I strive for perfection each and every day and to give back in some form. The question is often posed of what changed me. What made me turn it all around? To answer that, I always say being taken out of my environment and placed somewhere that was totally unfamiliar gave me an opportunity to see more and want more.

When I first moved to Florida, I was angry with everyone. But moving to Florida gave me an opportunity to see a different life. It is very difficult when a child is sent to detention and then released back into the same environment that put them there. Detention does not teach a child anything except how to build a thicker layer of skin, because it is about surviving. Some of the things that I learned in detention made me that much more street savvy. I learned in detention about how much money I could make by drug trafficking and how to use the coffee beans so that the dogs won't smell it! Most of us who are in trouble with the law and who are making bad decisions are not leaders, so we generally will not have the willpower to say no to drugs or other temptations that await us back in our same neighborhoods that we are released to. In addition, most of us are released back to the same drug-addicted families that contributed to us being where we are. I also have to say that having two mothers who loved me unconditionally through all my mess contributed in a major way to the changes that took place in me, but again they were one of a kind. Neither one of them ever dreamed of being a foster parent, but they changed their whole life plan for me. Most kids are not that fortunate, because most of the foster parents that we encounter today don't have patience with their own kids let alone someone else's. I see foster parents give up on children all the time because they curse them out, or they don't appreciate anything, or because they ran away. News flash: it is not about you! Of course they are going to take their anger out on you, but it is not about you; your job is to love them, and if you can't love them, don't add to the pain and neglect that they already feel.

The other sad part is that some children will be placed with foster parents who just don't care. So they never learn discipline and they never have structure. The foster parent does not care because it is just a paycheck. I urge all foster parents to please reevaluate and assess the reason why they became a foster parent. Don't cause more damage! Take the kids on trips out of town and show them things that they may never see. Read to them and help them develop study habits. And most of all, hold them accountable and don't back down when they rebel, because change is a process that does not occur overnight. I urge you to think about how you would feel and what you would do if you were abused and misused and then made to live with someone you don't know. Would you be friendly? Sometimes portraying an image of a bad ass is all we know how to do.

And last but not least, it is my belief in God and the plans that I know he has for my life that has set me free! I know that not everyone will have a relationship with God, but one thing I do know, is that I trust the plans he has for me, so when the storms come, I can stand strong and say, "Bring your best shot, devil, because I am always armed and ready to do spiritual warfare!" I now laugh in the face of the enemy. There is no way that I made it through all the hell that I have been through except to give back and to break the yoke of another wounded child or woman.

My sister and I are like night and day, and I believe that to be because she was not awarded the same opportunities as I. She was never taken out of her environment and awarded the opportunity to see something different. She looked for love in all the wrong places, and in return, she became a young mother who had no idea of how to parent a child because she never was parented. That is why we see so many young mothers in foster care; they are looking for someone to love them. But having a baby will never fill that void, especially when the father of the baby leaves you hanging dry. That will only add to your history of abandonment and set you further off course, because it will add to your years of anger. Also, I had to come to realize that it wasn't my mother or father who was hurting me, it was the drugs. Crack cocaine is a terrible drug, and it will continue to destroy our community. But we have to realize that we don't have to be our parents, and we can do more. We have the power to break generational curses! I may never have a relationship with my biological mother or father like a child deserves to, but I can now live a life where I am not as bitter, because I have a greater understanding of what drugs do to your mind.

Sometimes, I wish that more services were offered to my mom and dad to help them get off drugs, but I have no regrets about my life. I am happy that I went through what I did, because it has made me into the person that I am today! Now don't get me wrong I will always have wounds, but no one or nothing can break me! When I realized that I could have more, that I could go to college, and that I could own a house and help other people and children who were not as strong, I got a determination in me to help others! I have realized that actually working in this field is not for me. God has called me higher. When working in this field, your voice is often suppressed out of fear of losing your job or someone using your past against you and saying that you are too emotionally involved. My question is, why is not okay to love a child who has never been loved? The people who work with these kids are the best people to adopt and provide homes. All children need permanency and a place that will be their home even when they are twenty-one and no longer in the system, or forty-one; they still need a home. They will always need a family. When this book is read, I want people to know that despite what life may sometimes send your way, you are more than a conqueror, and trials only come to make you strong.

I am stronger today than I have ever been in my life. Many people said that I would not make it, and I remember having nightmares about being sentenced to life in prison for killing someone because I was so angry and bitter. There will never be enough words for the people who loved me through all my pain and saw something different in me when I did not even see it in myself. I have always been different, with my weird hair colors and my many tattoos, but all people are created differently. One thing that I tell all youth that I work with is there is a time and place for everything and never be afraid to be who God has called you to be. You are unique, and if I can do it, you can, too!

This book is a condensed version of my life. Some things I will never tell and some are to painful to mention. I have lived so many places and done so many things, but through it all, I look back and say thank you to everyone who played a part, even to the rotten apples—and there were many rotten apples! Remember: **what does not kill you will only make you strong**! When you decide to make a change for the better, you will begin to weed out some people who never meant you any good. Let them go, and as much as it hurts, don't try to make them stay.

As a foster parent, my prayer is that God helps me help every child who is entrusted to me. In helping them, I am helping myself. When I first became a foster parent, I was not ready. I was still angry and did not have a lot of patience. So God saw fit to take everything from me so that he could have one-on-one time with me, so that he could work on me. I thank him for that, because I am now able to love the way that I am supposed to, and I understand the importance of having balance.

Angel Bartlett

I ask all judges to please be involved and hold GALs accountable. Social workers hold futures in their hands. Probation officers, you also play a vital role in the success of the kids that are entrusted to you. So I admonish everyone to think harder and know that it is okay to go outside the box in order to assure that another child does not slip through the cracks.

In closing

In writing this book the devil has attacked me in many ways. My last two years of graduate school I lost Pastor Eddie, Self/Chip, and Mom Rigell. I got married and shortly after my marriage my husband/best friend cheated on me, he left me with a four hundred thousand dollar home and a daughter asking questions. I went into a deep dark depression. I was almost kicked out of school and I had to resign on several boards that I was a member of because I could not function. I had to send my daughter with her father because my depression was consuming my mind, body and spirit. I was too ashamed to talk with anyone so I could not ask for help or prayer. I contemplated killing my husband and calculated my every step. I was at a place where I felt like I had nothing to live for and my whole life flashed before me. It was in the darkest moment of my life when the Holy Spirit Spoke to me and said "WOUNDED, BUT NOT BROKEN". It is only a test and you will not fail, rise my child and seek me in the morning, noon and night. At that very moment I cried out and I praised the Most High like I had never praised him before! I learned to tarry all by myself! From that point I knew without a shadow of a doubt that the enemy could not steal anything from me. I had the power to possess the land. And at that very moment I began writing again and this time I would not stop!

I miss you Michael and I pray for you daily. I n my heart you are a lost person, but I believe that you will be found and that story is not finished! We were two broken people trying to love each other! I forgive you and my-self and I will always love you. I am always a phone call away. Remember prayer changes things!

To my grandma Daisy, I still have my mother living in you. To the entire Tose family, thank you for loving me and accepting me as family. To the Pettaway family, thank you for loving me even when I was crazy! To Ju-Ju and Self you may be gone, but never forgotten! To my cousin Q, thank you for leaving the streets alone. I promise we are going to see the overflow. To my Resurrection family, thank you for tarrying with me and the seeds that have been implanted deep in my heart! To Beth Stinnett, thank you for allowing me to have a voice and believing in me and also thank you for all the work that you do training people on alternatives to detention. Judge Dugger, I have never met a judge like you, but I can appreciate your passion. Those little talks that you have with children mean a lot. No matter how much you see them in your court, always remember that they are listening. To Hampton Social Services, thank you for allowing me to fulfill my dream of becoming a social worker! To everyone who said that I would never make it, I am still here, standing strong. I say that a lot in this book, because you will not believe the number of people who gave up on me at a young age, as if to say, "Suck up the abuse and get over it and live life normally." But it is not that easy, and you will never know that until you walk these shoes.

The same people who told me that would have never survived if they had to endure the things that I had to. *I am the strongest woman in the world!* To all the people who abused me and did not give me a chance to love, may God have mercy on your soul on judgment day! To all the other kids I met while in detention or in foster care, but somehow with all the different placements and constant moves we lost touch, I love you and I pray for you every day! To Counselor White and Counselor Rob, I pray that one day we can meet again so that you will know that I survived and I am doing very well! Thank you for locking me down in that holding cell when my temper got out of hand. You taught me lots of discipline!

To Crater detention, Christiansburg detention, Chesterfield detention, Henrico detention, Loundan County detention, Newport News detention, and Bon Air: here is a child who visited these places several times throughout my childhood, but I am here today and doing exceptionally well. Detention was my home away from home, but I still made it. So, when you look at some of those angry, disrespectful kids, think of me and what they have the potential to become. Be their biggest cheerleader, because sometimes you may be all they will ever have to speak a positive word of encouragement to them. Some of my counselors from detention were my best cheerleaders!

To Jessica Vermont, you were the realist social worker that I ever had; I thank you for your continued support! And to all my family and friends that I lost to the streets and to jail, you may be gone but never forgotten! To all my loved ones who got locked up as a juvenile and society never gave you a chance to make things right before they locked you up and threw away the key, I am and will always be your voice. And to James City County Department of Social Services, I say thank you and forgive me for all the hell that I put many of you through. Remember, you were working with someone who was wounded but not broken. To my sister, there is so much more that God has for you! To Mr. and Mrs. LaVille, thanks for being wonderful grandparents to my daughter. You are giving her all that I never had! Thank you. To Juanita

Bynum, Joyce Meyers, Mary j. Blige and Oprah Winfrey, I have never had the opportunity to meet you, but you have inspired, encouraged and uplifted me from a distance. I thank God for you women!

My mom Gwen always said that I would go from my GED to my PhD, and though she is not here today, I know she is looking down, smiling upon me. I miss you more than words can ever say. Thank you for loving me through my pain. To anyone I may have forgotten, please charge it to the head and not the heart, because marijuana really does kill your brain cells! ***Remember through all your mess there comes your message, and there is no testimony without the test! I forgive everyone that has ever hurt me.***

Scripts from my Past, and Present

On April 22, 1996, this worker visited the residence and learned from Angel that she had been picked up last night for curfew violation and that her father had picked her up from the police station. She again was not in school as she was wheezing in that she has asthma. Worker requested that Angel come with worker in order to receive medical attention, but Angel declined. Worker requested that if she went into distress to go to the emergency room immediately.

On April 23, 1996, we received a report at 2:30 A.M. from the hospital that Angel was in the emergency room and requested verbal permission to treat her. A decision was pending as to whether to hospitalize her. Social Worker Dallman and Charlton arrived at the hospital and learned that an alcohol screen had come back on Angel in that her alcohol level was at .98 and that she was intoxicated. Angel became disorderly and began yelling and cursing obscenities at hospital staff. The police were called to the scene and before they arrived Angel and a group of other teenagers who were at the hospital ran prior to the police's arrival.

The child's father provided minimal supervision to her and was not motivated to pursue family reunification. At this time her father is not an option and has directly influenced this child's lack of success. Angel's father is a substance abuser and previously had been ordered by his probation officer to enroll in a substance abuse program.

The child was removed from her mother's custody by the King & Queen Social Services and placed with her father in James City County. There has been some court intervention from the James City County Court ordering that the mother enroll and complete a substance abuse program. The child's mother has stated emphatically that she has no plans to stop using drugs and accepts no responsibility as to why the children are in foster care. Furthermore, she has no plans to ever resume any caretaking responsibilities of Angel.

3. **Briefly state child's situation, at the time placement occurred or custody is transferred. Information relative to family, health, education, must be addressed.**
At the time legal custody was transferred, _____, Angel's father, had disappeared while facing felony drug charges. The James City County Division of Social Services and the Juvenile Court Services Unit had attempted to work with Angel's mother, _____ who was unwilling to cooperate with the necessary services and therefore, could not be considered for a placement. Angel's health at that time was good and at the time she was in the eight grade.

Angel Bartlett

On April 22, 1996 we received a letter from Angel's therapist who expressed grave concern for Angel's safety in that she had received information from   , that Angel is selling drugs and is playing with guns and that she is doing whatever she wants.   has expressed concern for the safety of herself and her baby because of the crowd that Angel has begun to associate with. The therapist has recommended that a more structured environment be made available to Angel for her own safety. However, we have been unable to locate a facility who will accept Angel to include, Rosie Grier, Seton House, The Greenhouse less secure detention center and several others because of her aggressive tendencies.

You letter characterizes Angel has a troubled child with a lengthy criminal history and a troubled past, which she is. I remain concerned about the credence being given to statements by Angel that Virginia just wants to be "rid of her". Ms. Robinson and this agency have used all available resources and expended tremendous amounts of time and energy to get Angel to the only foster placement we felt could achieve some permanency. The Judge that has heard Angel's case since her original placement in foster care has said that he will not return her to either parent, ever. Both parents have long histories of alcohol and crack cocaine addiction and an unwillingness to address these issues. There is no relative willing to have Angel live with them under any circumstances.

Angel has been placed with every family member that could possibly take Angel and she has been removed at the relatives request. The community has paid for two therapeutic foster home placements, emergency shelters, intensive in home services for every placement that she has been in, and spent hours trying to locate Angel while she was on runaway status. (Which frequently over the last two years has been large chunks of time) Last year every attempt was made to support her father in attempting to regain custody of Angel by providing substance abuse treatment for the father, relocating the family to suitable housing, providing purchased services through a private company to offer intensive in home family therapy and an individual therapists for Angel.

Angel had been in ten different placements, including two commitments to the Department of Youth & Family Services, before she was placed in the home of The Rigell's. She is of considerable distance from her family and at the last court hearing on May 9, 1996, Judge Hoover stated that   is no longer an option for this child.

On January 16, 1996 Angel with was placed in her father's home. She was also assigned an individual therapist to work with her one on one within her home. She has made her self unavailable to these services.

On January 17, 1996 according to the agency security guard, Angel came into the agency under the influence of marijuana. The security guard indicated that Angel had a very strong and pronounced smell of marijuana in her clothing. This information was shared with her probation officer.

On February 14, 1996 Angel was admitted to Lafayette High school in their on-site alternative education program. She had limited success in that she was suspended three times within 40 days. At this time the school is recommending an alternative education placement for her. The acts committed at school include:

1) Simple Assault/Threatening
2) Inflammatory Actions/Harassment
3) Disrespect/ Defiance of School Staff's Authority
4) Unexcused Absences
5) General School and Classroom Disruption

In addition, Angel's boyfriend was involved in the shooting/gun incident that occurred at Lafayette High School. Once Angel was made aware that her boyfriend was involved she left the school premises without permission in order to locate him. In fact there have been two instances whereby she left school property without permission.

At this time the school officials are unwilling to accept her even in their off-site alternative education program. However, Angel is being allowed to attend school until the court could act upon the recommendations which is to request the court to order her to attend PMI or Enterprise Academy in Newport News. Angel opted instead not to return to school at all.

On February 29, 1996 Angel was verbally informed that she was released from probation. This Social Worker met with Barbara Ferrier on this date and informed her of the situation and the events that had occurred. This worker was told by Mrs. Ferrier that since there had been no new charges against Angel there was no reason to continue her on probation.

In March 1996 there was a shoot-out that occurred at New hope Park involving Angel and her friends. (This information was provided to this worker by the in home therapist) There was a teenager who was shot in the arm and hospitalized.

Information provided by :   was that Angel's boyfriend had put a gun to someones head.

Wounded, But Not Broken

ADDENDUM

NAME: Angel Bartlett DOB:02-10-81
JUDGE: Thomas B. Hoover
ATTORNEY: Mr. Dwight Dansby
ADDRESS: 6151 Centerville Rd, Williamsburg, VA 23188
COMMONWEALTH ATTORNEY: Mr. Pat Kelley
COUNSELOR: Sandra Diggs-Miller
COURT DATE: October 11, 1994

Angel Bartlett first came to the attention of the Court Service Unit in June of 1993 because of a fight she was involved in at Toano Middle School. At that time she was living in the Grove area of James City County with her father, , her sister, , and , a family friend. Subsequently, Angel was involved in two more fights on September 19, 1993 and October 15, 1993 before she finally had a dispositional hearing on February 8, 1994 when she was placed on probation. Her assigned probation counselor was Sandra Diggs-Miller.

Because structure in household was very loose, Angel still encountered problems and a protective service complaint was filed with James City County Social Services. There were allegations that cocaine was being openly sold from this household and that there were suspicions that the two girls were also involved. Additional problems encountered by Angel were in the form of missed probation appointments, staying out late or not coming home at all, and truancy. As a result, Angel was charged with violation of probation and she was detained. At the same time, James City County Social Services decided to refer Angel to the FAP Team and consideration was made to place Angel in a Lutheran Services Foster home.

On April 19, 1994, it was reported that Angel's father, , had left them and moved to Hampton, leaving no forwarding address. As a result, the Social Services Bureau was able to place Angel in Foster Care with the family of a girlfriend of Angel's. The plan was for her to stay in the home of Nancy Wagley until such time as she could be placed in a Lutheran Home. Unfortunately, this placement lasted only about two weeks and she was moved to the home of Gwen Rigall, who is the Assistant Principal at James Blair Intermediate School. That move was made on May 3, 1994 but only lasted for one week before she went AWOL and was placed back in detention on a charge of violation of probation.

On May 18, 1994, Angel was admitted to the Lutheran Home. This placement proved to be a more stable and supportive one in spite of the fact that Angel was not happy being there. The Social Service Bureau indicated that perhaps if an appropriate family member could be located that it would be a more suitable placement from a long term standpoint. Social Services was able to locate Mr. , Angel's maternal grandfather who, after some coaxing, agreed to try Angel at his home, and on August 17, 1994, that placement was completed. To supplement this placement it was also agreed that Lutheran Home Services would provide a counselor to work with Angel in the home to help her adjust to the new surroundings, and to help Mr. Bartlett and his paramour, , in coping with Angel.

Initially, this placement seemed doomed because almost immediately, Angel began

INITIAL ASSESSMENT

NAME: ANGEL BARTLETT

RACE: AFRICAN-AMERICAN

Angel initially came into the legal custody of The James City County Division of Social Services on January 24, 1995, after her maternal grandfather, _____, petitioned the court to be released of her custody. _____ had served as a custodian to Angel for only a brief period because she had been abandoned by her father.

On March 7, 1995, Angel was committed to the Department of Youth & Family Services and her foster care case was closed on that date. Upon her release from The Bon Air Juvenile Corrections facility, on May 11, 1995 the case was re-opened and Angel was placed in a therapeutic foster home.

On October 28, 1995, Angel ran away from her foster home and continued to involve herself in criminal activity. Angel was later apprehended in an abandoned house in Newport News by that police department on December 17, 1995. It had been learned that Angel was involved in gunfire exchange on the highway, but left the scene prior to her capture. There were no charges in regard to this matter, however her sister, _____, who also is in foster care, was apprehended and taken into police custody. Angel was placed in a detention center until her violation of parole hearing on January 16, 1996.

On January 16, 1996, Angel was placed in the home of her father, _____ and intensive home services were begun in order to provide stabilization and support services to the family. The family had two therapist working in the home with an individual therapist assigned to work with Angel.

After a few months it was apparent that her father was not willing to provide the level of care and supervision that Angel required and so she continued to involve herself with gang activity, drug use and weapons. The in-home therapist became increasingly concerned about the family's safety as _____ was spending very little time in the home and Angel again was in the midst of gunplay. The therapist recommended that Angel be removed from the home for her own safety.

Angel was placed in a relative home and St. Joseph's Villa for a brief period until the agency's CHINS petition was heard by the court as Angel was beyond Agency control in that she was not going to school, she was using drugs, she was involved in gunplay and in general continued to involve herself in criminal activities.

-On May 7, 1996 an order was entered which adjudicated Angel delinquent and a child in need of services. Angel was court ordered to refrain from the use of threatening and abusive behavior; that she cooperate with her therapist; that she enroll and attend school every day at the Peninsula Marine Institute; that she enroll in an anger management program; and that she enroll in a substance abuse program.

RECOMMENDATIONS:

Angel appears to be in need of long-term treatment services and a supportive environment to help her develop a positive identity for herself. She would likely benefit from learning anger management and problem solving skills, as well as relaxation techniques. Educational services focussing on substance abuse and sexually transmitted diseases is appropriate. Special education services for emotionally disturbed youth may need to be considered if Angel's emotional difficulties and low-frustration tolerance interfere with her being able to function in a regular classroom setting. Long-term individual therapy following her release into the community appears paramount as this youth needs to form a positive relationship with an adult. Her parole placement needs to be considered carefully. Finding an ideal placement will likely be difficult, but a facility which provides therapeutic services may be the most beneficial and least threatening for Angel. Angel's tendency to sabotage her relationships with others also needs to be considered when finding a placement. A referral for a psychiatric evaluation was made by this evaluator, and Angel may need to be monitored for further psychiatric services.

Jane Kudlas, Ph.D.
Resident in Psychology

Date of Evaluation: 3/27/95
Date Report Typed: 3/30/95

BEHAVIORAL OBSERVATIONS:

Angel was observed to be an attractive youth who physically appeared to be older than 14 years of age. Speech was often rapid and rambling, with Angel providing excessive detail or making tangential statements. When not speaking too quickly, she was easily understood. Mood appeared to vacillate, but Angel generally appeared angry or sullen. She was easily frustrated during the intellectual assessment, particularly during the Block Design and Object Assembly subtests of the WISC-III. At one point, she slammed the block on the desk. Upon inquiry, Angel indicated that she had difficulty concentrating because she was just thinking about throwing the test material. Fortunately, Angel responded to praise and encouragement and seemed to do better when she was informed about what the task would entail. She followed directions and put forth good effort despite her level of frustration.

High levels of anger, depression, and anxiety were reported. Although current suicidal ideation was denied, Angel said she had contemplated killing herself in the past. Angel also noted that she no longer has homicidal thoughts, but said she once planned on killing her mother. Angel indicated that she was afraid of her anger, mentioning that she will not allow herself to be alone with her sister's children for fear of getting annoyed and then "throttling" or shaking them too hard. Angel noted difficulties getting and staying asleep since her incarceration, and she reported a poor appetite. She also noted intrusive thoughts or flashbacks concerning the abuse she and her sister experienced. Crying spells were also reported. Negative feelings and thoughts were noted to occur when alone. Hallucinations were denied, and delusional thinking was not evident. Angel was clearly oriented to person, place, and time.

Personality testing is reflective of a significantly depressed and angry youth who feels inadequate in managing her environment and her own emotions. Problems controlling her anger contribute to feelings of anxiety and nervousness, as well as damage Angel's already low self-image. Angel shows some insight into her angry feelings and appears to be using cognitive resource to keep herself from acting on these feelings, but her resources are limited and Angel is likely to have difficulty containing aggressive impulses, particularly in unstructured, stressful situations. Angel appears to have difficulty utilizing resources in a coherent fashion which may contribute to unpredictable acting-out behaviors or displays of affective discontrol.

Although this youth is not psychotic, testing suggests that her reality-testing becomes tenuous in times of emotional distress. Failure to attend to various cues and a tendency to base perceptions on small pieces of information appears to effect her ability to make good decisions or even be aware of problems that need attention. Additionally, her high level of emotional distress often contributes to her trying to avoid difficult situations. Thus, she not only fails to solve problems, but she also makes her situation worse by creating additional difficulties in her attempts to avoid the initial problem.

Even though Angel is extremely needy and constantly seeks attention in inappropriate ways, she remains emotionally distant. She fears rejection and abandonment, while also engaging in behaviors which confirm her fears. Poor interpersonal relations, in turn, contributes to Angel's anger and depression and likely promotes her attention seeking behaviors. Testing suggests severely damaged

Wounded, But Not Broken

Ms. Menke picked up Angel at the airport on 9-19-96. Angel did not have anything except the clothes that she was wearing and a bag with candy in it. She did not have a toothbrush, comb, deodorant, feminine hygiene products or clothes (including underclothes). She did have the letter guaranteeing payment from Virginia, ICPC 100-B and a medical release. They had to go out that night and purchase items that Angel could sleep in and also for the morning so that she did not have to put on the same clothes (sweat pants) that she was wearing when she arrived. Ms. Menke received an AirborneExpress package on 9-23-96 containing medical and education information about Angel. She still needed court work and the licensing problem addressed. A copy of the educational information was taken to Mrs. Rigell. Angel has not been in any school long enough to earn credits for over a year. Mrs. Rigell is a Principal and Educator in Sarasota so she was able to help with an educational direction for Angel. Angel has seemed to self-educate herself. Her reading and writing skills far surpass her educational training. On 9-24-96 Ms. Menke called Ms. Robinson again requesting the court work be sent. Court work varies from state to state so they agreed on her sending anything signed by a judge. Ms. Menke asked if she had mailed clothing allowance check or clothing in her office yet. She stated that she had requested a check be cut but could not control this time frame. She earlier had promised both Mrs. Rigell and Ms. Menke that the check would be sent Federal Express. She stated that she had not been able to find a box to mail Angel's clothes and had been very busy.

NAME: ANGEL BARTLETT   DOB: 02/10/81   SC#: 48202   R/S: B F

VII. PSYCHOLOGICAL INFORMATION:

relations with both parents, and a view that relationships are conflictual and hostile. Although Angel appears to have some empathy skills, she is generally too needy and too self-engrossed to be concerned with the needs of others. Problems with relations are likely to be a long-term concern for this youth who appears to be developing a Borderline Personality Disorder.

Angel Bartlett

COMMUNITY SERVICE

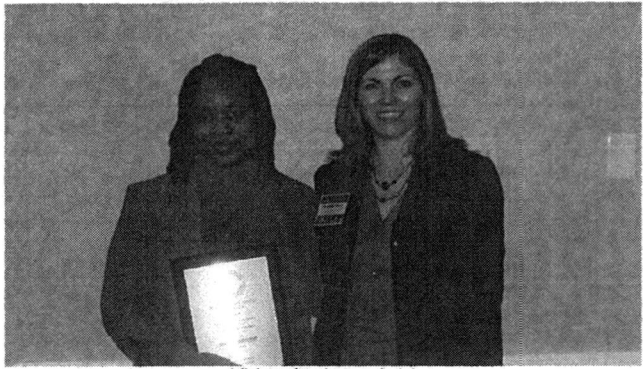

(click to view larger photo)

ANGEL BARTLETT
2008 Meritorious Award Winner
in the Area of Community Service
(Pictured with VJJA President Beth Stinnett)

"For those who entered the field of juvenile justice believing that people can change, and that despite getting off to a rough start children involved in the delinquency system can grown into positive and productive young adults, this recipient is a living testament and a reminder most children age out of delinquent behavior and that children are not yet who they will become.

A former foster care child, probationer, and resident of Bon Air Juvenile Correctional Center, our recipient is now a college graduate, a social worker, a youth advocate, a full-time graduate student, a homeowner, a biological and foster care parent – all of this by age 27.

Despite significant hurdles during childhood and adolescence, as a young adult our recipient has worked as a Family Crisis Stabilization Worker, assisting children and families experiencing the same challenges she once faced. A passionate advocate who leads with both her head and her heart, she has participated in the Hampton community's Juvenile Detention Alternatives Initiative (JDAI) and has been a part of efforts to reduce an over-reliance on secure confinement and other out of home placements.

In June our recipient was named the 2008 Virginia Spirit of Youth award winner. The award recognizes and celebrates a young adult who has made great strides following involvement with the juvenile justice system; has overcome personal obstacles; and is making significant contributions to society. This summer she addressed a group of juvenile court judges at a national conference sponsored by the National Council of Juvenile and Family Court Judges. She

ANGEL

Mother
Student
Is what you chose,

Assignments
Internship
Brought many whoas!

Dreadlocks
Body art
Is what we see,

Spiritual
Afrocentric
How expressed thee.

Zealous
Committed
A goal to prove,

Focused
Family oriented
Surely did do.

University
Graduate
It's been a whirl,

Master's degree
Social worker
GO ON GIRRRRL!

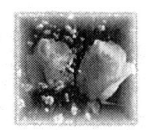

© Denise J. Hines

The Lord is my Shepherd. I shall not be in want.

He makes me lie down in green pastures, he leads me beside quiet waters, and he restores my soul.

He guides me in paths of righteousness for his names sake.

Even though I walk through the valley of the shadow of death
I WILL FEAR NO EVIL

For he is with me, his rod and his staff comfort me.

He prepares a table before me in the presence of my enemies.

He anoints my head with oil; my cup overflows.
Surely goodness and love will follow me all the days of my life, and I will dwell in the house of the LORD forever.
Psalm:23

To contact Angel please visit our website at:
www.Angelbartlett.com
and also look out for
"Wounded But Not Broken, Part 2"
"A Message to the Enemy"
"It Isn't Over"

Breinigsville, PA USA
24 August 2010
244116BV00001B/3/P